HEALING

Roots of Modern Orthopedic and Spine Surgery

How surgeons, businessmen, engineers and, yes, lawyers created the modern system of fixing hips, knees, spines and more.

By: Robin Young

Contributing writers: James Bradley, Journalist
Dr. Charles Crawford, Professor of History and Director of the Oral History Research Office at The University of Memphis.

Editor: Robin R. Young

First Edition

For information about special discounts for bulk purchases, please contact RRY Publications LLC at www.ryortho.com.

Title: Healing: The Roots of Modern Orthopedic and Spine Surgery

Description: First edition. | RRY Publications LLC

ISBN: 978-0-9779648-5-7

DEDICATION AND ACKNOLOWLEGMENT

This book would not have been possible without the substantial and consequential research and talented journalism of James Bradley, and Dr. Charles Crawford, Professor of History and Director of the Oral History Research Office at The University of Memphis. At his wife's urging, L.D. Beard sat down with James Bradley and Dr. Crawford to provide an oral history of Richards Manufacturing, Danek, Sofamor Danek and more. Also participating with L.D. Beard and his wife Betty Beard was Ron Pickard. The entire body of work by James Bradley and Dr. Crawford was compiled into a draft book titled: "As Far North as Memphis". This landmark work of oral history and academic research is also a superbly written account of a bygone era. It deserves to be read and I am both humbled and honored to be able to include portions of it in this book.

This book is also dedicated to Rick Treharne, Ph.D., Ron Pickard, Alan Olsen, Robert Compton, Randal Betz, M.D., Terry Stahurski, M.D., Seth Greenwald Ph.D., Rich Ashman, Ph.D., James Moran, Jules Falcone, Eric Muehlbauer, Stephen Phillips, Hansen Yuan, M.D., Alex Lukianov, Shawn McGuinn, Art Steffee, M.D. and, most especially, an engineer who had the great good fortune of being at the right place at the right time—multiple times. And who, for several years, held more patents than any other engineer at Medtronic, the second largest medical device company in the world. A mensch and dear friend of many decades; Michael Sherman.

Robin Young, 2022

Contents

INTRODUCTION 13

CHAPTER ONE: THE TAP ROOT OF MODERN ORTHOPEDICS 1784-1958 15

Orthopedics as Pediatric Deformity Correction Practice ... 16

The American Civil War 19

Hospital for Special Surgery is Founded 26

Early Hip Surgery 27

Unexpected Breakthrough: The First Hip Replacement 34

CHAPTER TWO: JOINT REPLACEMENT 38

From Dentistry to Orthopaedics 39

Forged in World War II 41

The Idea of a Total Hip Replacement Takes Root 42

Charnley Rejects Lubricating the Hip, Narrows the Problem 43

Charnley Goes Single-Cup and Excises the Femoral Head 44

Acrylic Dental Cement 45

Charles F. Thackray Ltd and Harry Craven Join Charnley 45

Craven Tests a New Plastic 47

Eureka! but Charnley Blocks Wide Distribution 48

Charnley Meets Seth Greenwald 50

Charnley, Müller and the AO 52

Charnley's Way or the Highway 56

CHAPTER THREE: THE PRACTICES OF SUPPLYING AND EDUCATING ORTHOPEDIC SURGEONS EMERGES IN WARSAW AND MEMPHIS 60

Revra DePuy 61

Justin Zimmer 63

AAOS Is Born and Modern Orthopaedics Takes Form in Memphis 65

Dr. Willis Cohoon Campbell – The First President of American Academy of Orthopaedic Surgeons (AAOS) 67

CHAPTER FOUR: RICHARDS MANUFACTURING 73

Harry Treace 77

Leander Dallas Beard 80

Firestone Tire and Rubber 88

The U.S. Air Force 91

L.D. Finds His Way to Richards Manufacturing. 93

Creating the First Orthopaedic Device Packaging Line 98

Creating a Medical Inventory and Shipping Operations System From Scratch 99

Don Richards Dies Unexpectedly 99

Union 101

CHAPTER FIVE: ORTHOPEDIC MANUFACTURING BECOMES A GROWTH INDUSTRY 104

The Stanmore Group 108

The Redhill-Ring Group 110

The Exeter Group 113

Hard Choices 116

Making the Devices 116

Zimmer UK 117

Down Brothers 120

Deloro Stellite 121

Howmedica 121

Zimmer USA 123

DePuy 123

Orthopaedics Accelerates Dramatically and Richards New Team Finds Its Rhythm 126

Medicare Becomes Rocket Fuel for Orthopaedic Growth 131

CHAPTER SIX: NAPKIN DRAWINGS, INNOVATION, MEMPHIS, MANUFACTURING, WARSAW 139

Rorer 143

New Owners, New Products, and a Diffusion of Focus 144

Hips, Knees and So Much More 146

The Modular Knee Innovation 151

Comfort Care 152

CHAPTER SEVEN: RON PICKARD: THE MOST CONSEQUENTIAL MANAGER OF THEM ALL 157

Leaving Comfort Care 163

Pickard Moves Up the Ranks 166

CHAPTER EIGHT: THE ILLIZAROV EXTERNAL FRAME 170

Dr. Dror Paley 174

The Illizarov External Fixator Project Accelerates 175

Bridging the Cultural Divide Between Russia, Illizarov and America's Ortho Entrepreneurs 178

Playing the Winner's Game in Orthopaedics 179

The First Course in Kurgan, Siberia 184

CHAPTER NINE: FDA, ASTM AND THE ORTHOPAEDIC SURGICAL MANUFACTURER ASSOCIATION 187

The FDA Becomes a Power Player in Orthopaedics in 1986 189
Preemption of State Laws 192
Big Changes at Richards 194
Treace Is Replaced, L.D. Beard Becomes President 198
CHAPTER TEN: SPINE SURGERY BECOMES A SPECIALTY 202
The Beginning of Modern Spine Surgery 204
Karl Alfred, Arthur Steffee, and Dennis Stuart 204
Testing, Training and Fabrication 206
Spinning Ideas and Concepts 207
Fabricating an Implant for Steffee *DURING* Surgery 209
The First Implanted Artificial Human Vertebrae 210
The End of CRI 214
The Fire 217
Hard Choices 218
Danek 220
The Luque Screw 223
CHAPTER ELEVEN: FROM COTREL TO TSRH ... 229
Abe Glasser, Stuart Medical and the One and Only Julius Falcon 233
Alan Olsen Meets Eduardo Luque 239
Texas Scottish Rite Hospital 241
Ron Pickard Leaves Richards, Joins Beard and Alan Olson at Danek 247
Funding a Start-Up in a New Medical Specialty .. 249
Robert Compton 250

A Million Dollars for...Hardware? 251
Going Public 254
The Nine Month IPO Delay 255
"The Spine Specialist" 257
Buying Yves Cotrel's Sofamor 258
The Sofamor Deal Goes on Life Support – Twice 260
Who's Name Goes First? 261
The End of Spine at Stuart Medical 262
The Effect of Sofamor on Danek 263
Safe Medical Devices Act of 1990 264
CHAPTER TWELVE: 1993 – BEST OF TIMES AND WORST OF TIMES 266
A Public Attack on Fixation Screws in Spine Surgery 269
Putting Malpractice Liability on the Manufacturer 273
"You're Served" 275
TV Commentators and Public Opinion vs Scientific Evidence 277
The Mass Tort Playbook 280
"If you're right, you're right. And you've got to stick by that." 280
Don't Let the Other Side Get Between You and Your Customer 282
'Burn the Ships'—There Is No Turning Back 284
Jim Gallogly Takes Over as President and Chief Operating Officer 289
Wall Street Analysts 289
NASS, AAOS and Individual Surgeons Are Sued 290

How the Most Consequential Lawsuit in Medical History Was Won 293

Intended Use 294

The First Major Plaintiff Loss: Class Certification Denied 296

Judge Louis C. Bechtle Takes Charge 297

Attacking the "Defective Device" Claim 298

Phantom Cases 300

Separating FDA Myth From FDA Reality 301

Defending Spine Surgeon's Ability to Practice Medicine 303

Goofball "Experts" 304

Ending 1,200 Tennessee Lawsuits With a Single Letter 305

Game, Set, Match 308

The Toll 310

The Long-term Effect of the Pedicle Screw Litigation 311

Medtronic Buys Sofamor Danek for $1.7 Billion .. 313

CHAPTER FOURTEEN: THE GOLDEN AGE FOR ORTHOPEDICS AND SPINE 318

DePuy 319

1990s: DePuy Manufacturing Undergoes Diversification and Acquisitions 320

Zimmer 323

Bristol-Myers Buys Zimmer: 1970s-2000 324

Zimmer Holdings Is Spun Off and Goes Public. 326

Biomet 327

Dane's Tenacity 328

Biomet Culture 329

Dane: "They All Thought I Was Nuts" 329
Dane and Mary Louise 330
Fighting for the Team 331
Stryker Corporation 332
The Industry in 2022 335
The Largest Sector in Medicine 336
EPILOGUE 338

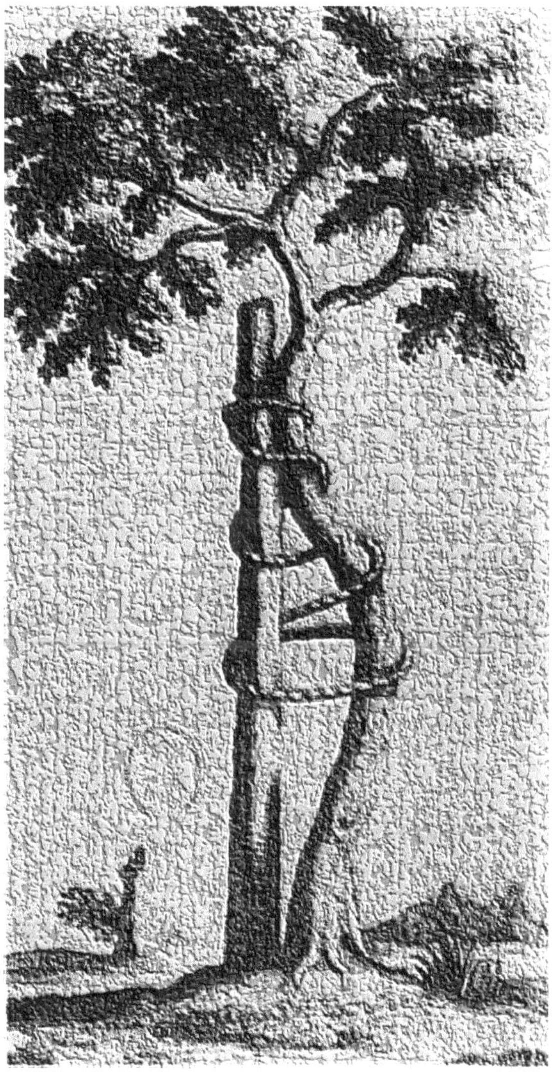

THE TORTUOUS PATH TO HIP ARTHROPLASTY

Early 19th Century
HENRY PARK: Treated hip deformity by excising the femoral head, basically performing excision hip arthroplasty.

1821
ANTHONY WHITE 1st excision arthroplasty on a 9-year old patient with hip tuberculoses. Also used in patients with infected hips.

1826
JOHN RHEA BARTON 1st osteotomy on an ankylosed hip. Demonstrated that motion could prevent fracture healing and bone formation.

1840
CARNOCHAN: Wood blocks for interposition arthroplasty

1854
LEWIS SAYRE: Resected hips in 59 patients, of which 39 survived (no anesthesia or sterile field)

1860
AUGSTUS STANISLAV: First soft tissue interposition arthroplasty

1880
LEOPOLD OLLIER Interposition of adipose tissue in aseptic joints.

1891
THEMISTOCLES GLUCK Made a ball and socket joint from ivory that was fixed to the bone with nickel plated screws

1896
VITEZSLAV CHLUMSKY, HEINRICH HELFERICH, ERICH LEXER, FOEDRE, WILLIAM STEVEN BAER Wide variety of interposition materials, such as muscle, celluloid, silver plates, rubber struts, magnesium, zinc, glass, pyres, decalcified bones and wax were tested on patients.

Early 20th Century
JOHN BENJAMIN MURPHY: Removed osteophytes around the articulating surfaces of the joint

1918
ROBERT JONES Gold foil to cover reconstructed femoral heads. 21-year follow-up showed good function and pain relief

1919
PIERRE DELBET Used rubber as a prothesis to replace joint surfaces

1923
MARIUS STEVEN-PETERSON Interposition arthroplasty using glass. Later substituted Vitallium and this resulted in the first predictable clinical outcomes for interpositional hip arthroplasty

1933
ERNEST W HEY-GROVES: Uses ivory as a prosthetic material to replace joint surfaces

1938
PHILLIP WILES First total hip arthroplasty using stainless steel components fitted to the bone with bolts and screws

1940's
EDWARD HARBUSH, KENNETH McKEE Uses dental acrylic cement as the fixation material to hold components in place.

1948
ROBERT AND JEAN JUDET Uses an acrylic prosthesis to replace joint surfaces

1950
FREDERICK ROECK THOMPSON Uses Vitallium as a material for prosthesis to replace stem and femoral head

1950-52
HAROLD BOHLMAN, AUSTIN MORE Created a Vitallium femoral sided implant which was refined to feature a fenestrated stem which allowed bony ingrowth.

1953
GEORGE MCKEE Uses a Vitallium femoral stem and a combination of cobalt chrome for the acetabular cup.

Late 1950s
JOHN CHARNLEY Invented low friction torque arthroplasty, use of acrylic cement to fix components to the bone and high density polyethylene as an articulating bearing surface

INTRODUCTION

Fixing arthritic, ankylosed, cancer ridden or traumatically fractured large joints was a tortuous medical and manufacturing journey.

It took 160 years to get to John Charnley in the 1950s. Then another four decades to get to modern orthopedics and spine.

The revolution of safe and successful procedures, instruments and implants took shape in the late 1950s and accelerated over the next 40 years. Many of the pioneers are still among us. Their stories are the backbone of this book.

In retrospect, the urgent imperative to heal—despite a lack of knowledge and tools—drove these pioneering surgeons, engineers, and manufacturers forward. Theories were tested. Advances came agonizingly slowly at first.

Today, every 3.6 seconds, a healthcare provider somewhere in the world employs techniques, uses instruments and/or man-made constructs which reach back to the ideas of these pioneering surgeons and engineers.

For patients around the world orthopedic surgery is little short of a miracle.

This book is the first in a series. It covers the underground part of a largely untold story—the roots.

Here is how the modern practice of fixing degenerative, diseased, or fractured musculoskeletal system took root and grew.

Robin Young December 2022

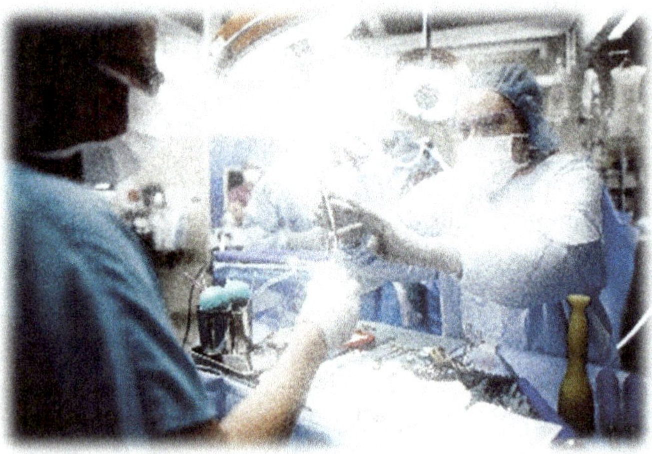

CHAPTER ONE: THE TAP ROOT OF MODERN ORTHOPEDICS 1784-1958

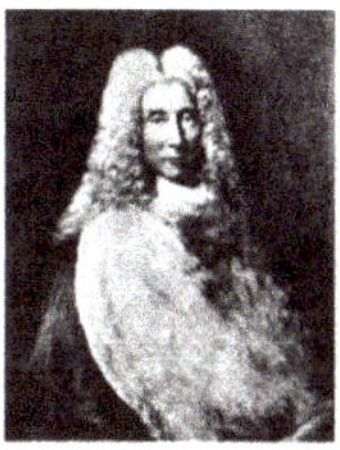

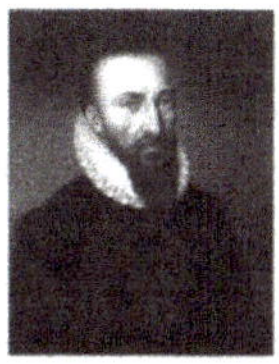

Ambroise Pare, author of *Ten Books of Surgery*

Nicolas Andry de Bois-Regard 1700s

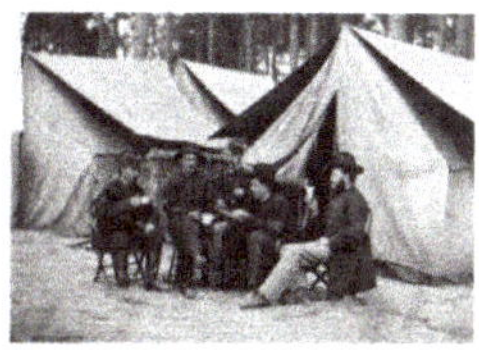

Civil War Surgeons in front of their tent

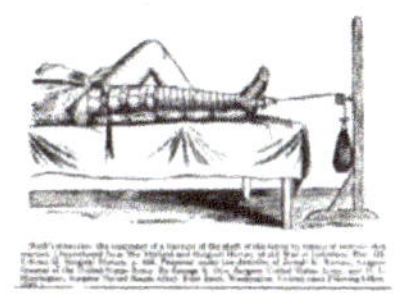

Buck's Traction

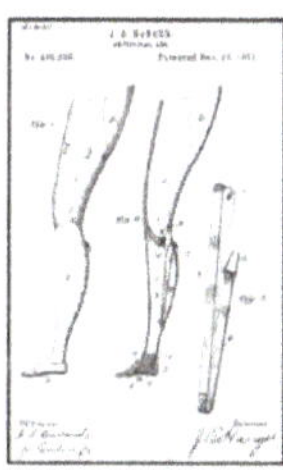

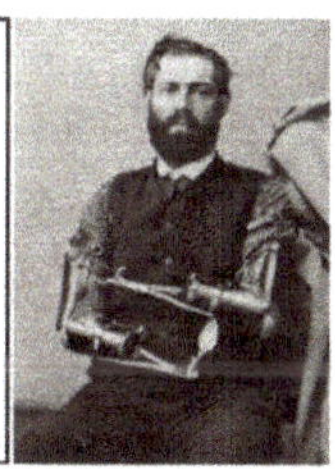

Civil War veteran, Samuel Decker, and his prosthetics

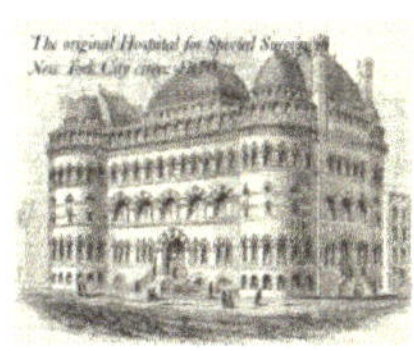

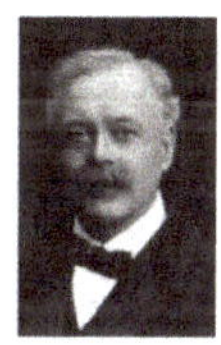

Robert Jones

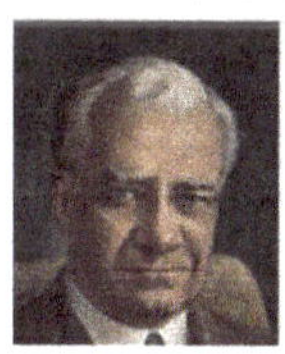

Marius Nygaard Smith-Petersen

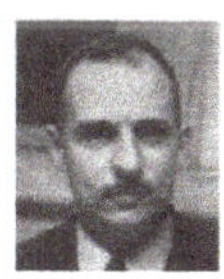

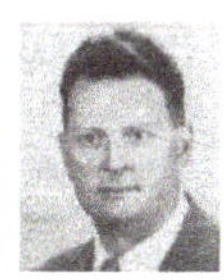

Robert and Jean Judet

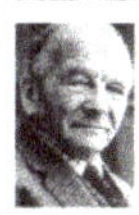

Dr. Kenneth McKee

The practice of orthopedic and spine surgery—the replacement of human bone and soft tissues with a man-made metals, plastics and other materials—is usually thought of as a recent development, a product of modern science, new technologies, and new materials. That view is only superficially correct.

Advances in science and medicine typically have far earlier beginnings and take longer, more tortuous roads than most people realize. For diseases, deformities and traumatic damage to the musculoskeletal system, nothing good happened overnight.

Indeed, each major advance seemed to require military conflict—for a while.

As late as 1950, medical implants were virtually unheard of among the general population, and orthopedic surgery was used mainly to treat severe bone fractures. "Hip surgery" was something surgeons did for broken hips. Immobile, arthritic hips were the disease of old age and therefore uncurable and treatable only with canes, wheelchairs and pain relief medicines including addictive opiates.

Joints simply wore out This had been true when the first medical texts were written, and it was still true in the mid-twentieth century—when technology and medicine were about to cross a major threshold together.

Orthopedics as Pediatric Deformity Correction Practice

The term *orthopedia* itself did not exist until 1741. That was the year Nicholas Andry de Bois-Regard, a professor of medicine at the University of Paris, used it as the title for his book describing "the different methods of preventing and correcting the deformities of children." He formed the word (in French, *orthopédie*) by combining the Greek words *ortho*, meaning straight or free from deformity, and *paidios*, meaning “child.” This reflected what was then the primary concern of physicians who treated skeletal problems: the correction of childhood deformities.

The causes of such conditions and related pain included not only birth defects and fractures, but osteomyelitis (an infection of the bone or bone marrow) and diseases such as polio and tuberculosis of the bones and joints.

In Andry’s time medical options were few: each disease or infection would run its usual course—vaccines and antibiotics lay far into the future—and subsequent treatments were limited to primitive corrective devices.

Where physicians could make a difference, however, was setting and stabilizing bone fractures through careful application of splints and traction devices, but even this approach had its limitations. If a complicated fracture required amputation or other major surgery, that lay beyond the skills and training of ordinary physicians. The reason for this was a division of labor that seems bizarre today: for centuries actual surgery was performed by barber-surgeons, not by physicians.

The practice of medicine was the province of physicians who relied principally on academic theory—but without benefit of the scientific method. That would come later.

The views of the second century Roman physician Galen still dominated medical theory. The medical profession of the day diagnosed and treated the patient non-intrusively. This professional divide probably developed in the Middle Ages for arcane religious and social reasons, but it continued on into the early years of the modern era.

Surgical advances did eventually find a way into hospitals and medical treatises, and by the 1500s a French surgeon, Ambrose Paré, could publish *Ten Books of Surgery*, a massive work that greatly improved the treatment of battlefield wounds and became a standard text for surgeons.

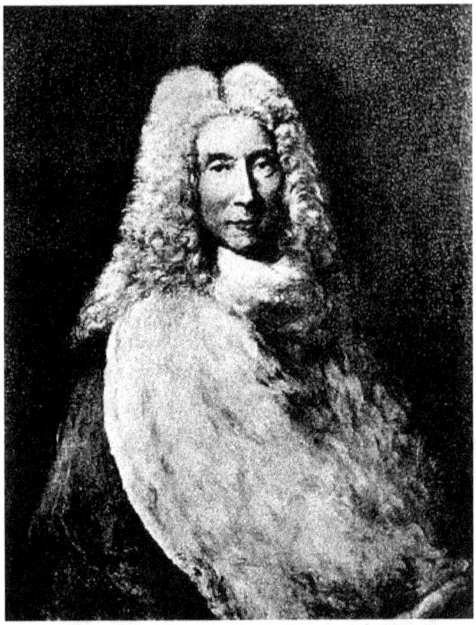

Nicolas Andry de Bois-Regard 1700s
Source: Wikipedia.com

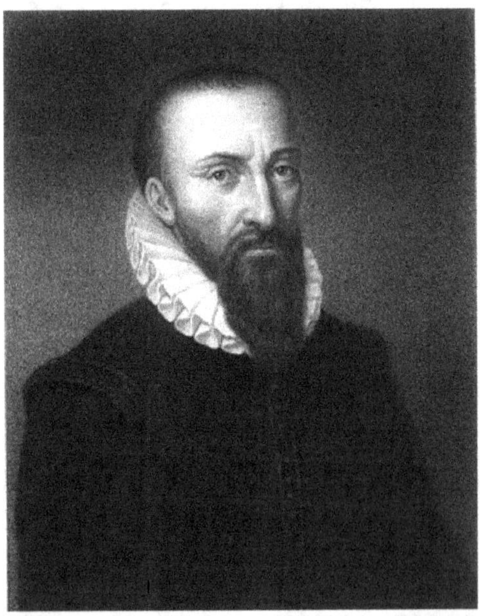

Ambrose Paré, author of Ten Books of Surgery
Source: Wikipedia.org

War had always meant broken bones and amputations of severely damaged limbs, but the instances of each multiplied after the appearance of cannons in the fourteenth century. Horrific wounds became commonplace (as did warfare, seemingly). Army surgeons were slow to develop new skills and techniques to address life-threatening injuries. Paré wanted to change that, and he is now credited with laying "the foundation upon which the modern institution of surgery is built."

As European wars came and went, the care and treatment of battlefield injuries continued to improve, as did the status of surgeons. So much so, in fact, that by the mid-eighteenth-century members of the relatively new Academy of Surgery in Paris were even accorded the same privileges as the Faculty of Medicine. With surgeons no longer regarded as mere technicians, traditional medicine and surgical skill began to overlap, if not actually join.

But progress in the field of orthopedic surgery was painfully slow. The Napoleonic Wars of the late eighteenth and early nineteenth century, with armies numbering in the tens of thousands, pushed battlefield medicine and surgical skills to their limits. And while the French army did develop a remarkably efficient medical service system for its time, the death rate in military hospitals in the last two years of Napoleon's reign hovered above 28%. It would take another war, fifty years later on another continent, to bring about some of the greatest surgical advances in the treatment of severe bone injuries.

The American Civil War

Orthopedic surgery in the United States had its origins in the American Civil War, a conflict in which advances in weaponry, especially in terms of the damage they could inflict upon the human body, had far outpaced medical skill and technology.

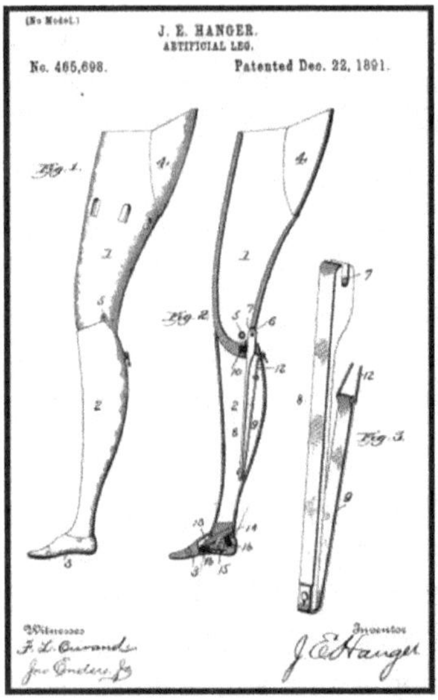

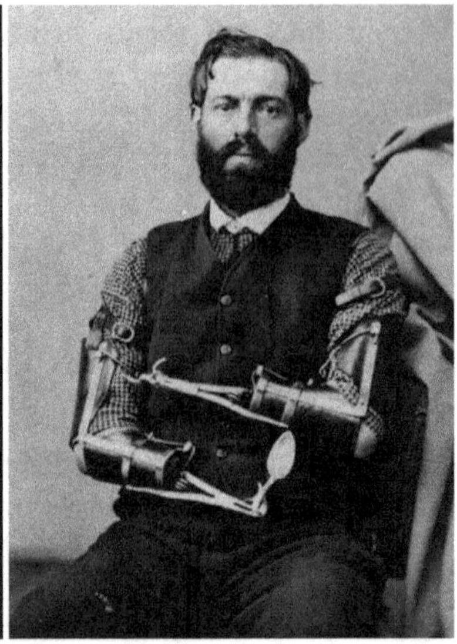

Civil War Veteran, Samuel Decker, and His Prosthetics

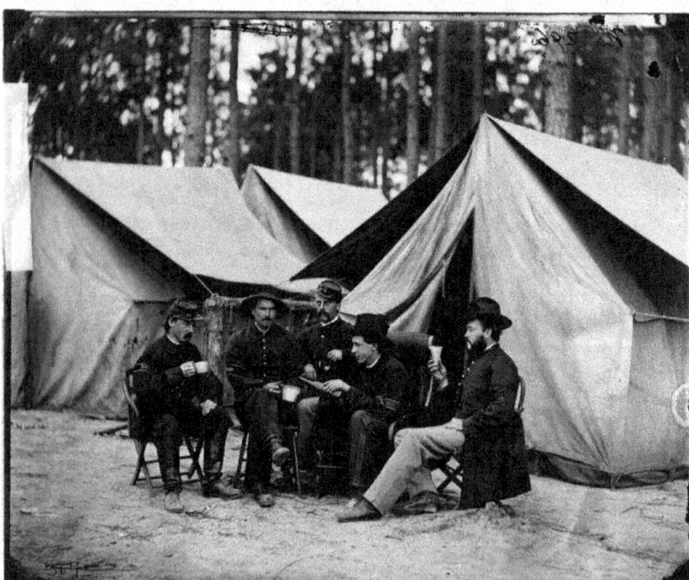

Civil War surgeons in front of their tent
Source: National Museum of Civil War Medicine

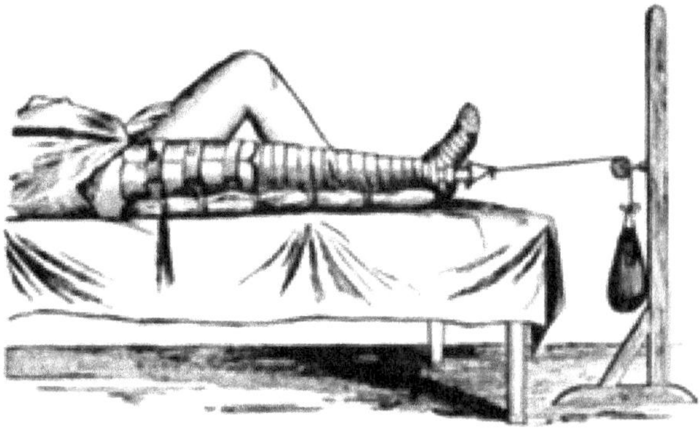

Buck's extension: the treatment of a fracture of the shaft of the femur by means of [illegible] skin traction. (Reproduced from The Medical and Surgical History of the War of Rebellion. Part III. Volume II, Surgical History, p. 348. Prepared under the direction of Joseph K. Barnes, Surgeon General of the United States Army. By George A. Otis, Surgeon United States Army, and [illegible] Huntington, Surgeon United States Army. First Issue. Washington, Government Printing Office, [illegible].)

Buck's Traction / Source: Springer Nature Switzerland AG

A common misconception is that Civil War surgeons routinely resorted to amputation of arms and legs when confronted with any compound fracture. The records show otherwise. Amputations were certainly common, but the treatments that were attempted were far more varied than this notion allows, and the large number of injuries presented surgeons with almost limitless opportunities to try new procedures or modify old ones in their efforts to save limbs and maximize patient rehabilitation afterwards.

Complicating every surgery was the risk of infection, which was often fatal. Although Joseph Lister's discoveries in antiseptics would not be published until after the Civil War, many medical practitioners had at least some idea of the causes of sepsis, commonly known as blood poisoning, and various antiseptic procedures were tried. Unfortunately, the niceties of sterilization frequently had to be overlooked on the battlefield or, sometimes still, were simply not regarded as essential.

Despite this, many army surgeons developed new ideas and techniques throughout the war, and the conflict brought about major improvements in the care of the wounded on both sides. It was also during the war that the American medical profession first began to specialize—doctors skilled in surgery were called "operators"—and this helped weed out inexperienced physicians and surgeons and those whose skills were unsuited to the procedures necessary to save joints and limbs.

Hospitals were quick to adopt the idea of specialization, especially in the South where the number of maimed soldiers returning home created a desperate need for specialized care.

The extent of this need is evidenced by an observation recorded by one postwar visitor to a southern town. While attending a public meeting in Aberdeen, Mississippi, he noticed that fully a third of the 300 or so men present had lost either an arm or a leg. Nor was Aberdeen unique. In the first year after the war ended, the State of Mississippi spent one-fifth of its entire revenue on artificial limbs.

Because the treatment of wounds varied greatly in the early days of the war, owing to the different experience levels of individual surgeons, each side developed manuals to improve and standardize medical care.

Medical *journals*, publications critical to information on new techniques and procedures, were another matter, and these were especially hard to find on the Confederate side. It was only towards the end of the Civil War that the *Confederate States Medical and Surgical Journal* was published and widely circulated, and by then it was too late to be a significant factor.

Even so, the lack of published journals in the South should not be taken as evidence of a lack of quality or knowledge by Confederate medical practitioners. Physicians and surgeons in each army would treat captured wounded soldiers as well as their own, and this often allowed them to see the work that surgeons on the other side had performed and to comment on it.

Reports show that Union surgeons were often surprised at the expertise of Confederate surgeons and the degree of difficulties they had overcome in certain procedures. Indeed, it appears that out of this grew a degree of mutual rivalry with each side trying to outdo the accomplishment of enemy surgeons, and the combination of sharing and competition actually enhanced the quality of care for wounded soldiers on both sides.

Also important to future orthopedic medicine—especially the lengthy surgeries that would be needed for medical implants—was the extensive use of anesthesia during the war. Despite the "biting-the-bullet" image frequently associated with the treatment of the wounded, it was relatively rare for Civil War soldiers to undergo surgery without any anesthesia whatsoever. Both chloroform and ether were available, each having first been used in surgeries during the Mexican War in 1847.

Of the two, chloroform became the anesthesia of choice because it was more accessible—a key factor especially in the South—and because it was more easily transportable and presented less of a fire hazard than ether. And the use of anesthesia was generally safe: less than one-half of one percent of all the patients to whom it was administered died as a direct result of the anesthesia itself. The use of opium in follow-up care to suppress pain also allowed more extensive surgical procedures to be conducted.

The kinds of fractures surgeons encountered varied greatly, although the majority of the injuries suffered on both sides of the conflict were wounds to extremities, a fact no doubt attributable to the effectiveness of the rifled musket and the recently developed minié ball. A bullet shot from an old smoothbore musket would typically break the bone upon impact, whereas the energy expended by the new weapons and ammunition would splinter, shatter, and split the bones.

Besides the extensiveness of the damage, other factors that influenced the decision as to whether to amputate or not included which extremity was involved and the wound's location—the nearer the break to the torso, the riskier the surgery.

It is probable that the high mortality rate (nearly 100%) associated with amputations due to wounds to the upper thigh meant that amputations in such instances were rare. As the war continued, surgeons became more conservative in their approach to treating wounds, with amputation becoming the least favored option.

Wounds to the shoulder and hip typically posed the greatest difficulties for surgeons because these injuries required repair of the joints themselves, a very complex and exacting procedure, and also because it was so difficult to keep the repaired joint immobilized. The most effective treatment for shoulder injuries was the surgical removal of part or parts of bone tissue—in medical parlance, "resection arthroplasty. It offered the best chance for retaining a functional limb. On the other hand, hip wounds produced the highest mortality rates, regardless of the method of treatment.

The conservative, and safest, treatment for hip injuries typically involved various traction devices, such as Buck's traction, variations of which are still widely used today.

Invented by a New York physician Gurdun Buck, his mechanism employed a system of ropes and weights that pulled or stretched the extremity to keep it immobilized during healing. Other devices were Smith's anterior splint (named for Nathan R. Smith), which suspended the leg from the ceiling, and Hodgen's splint, which was similar. Both used wire rods that could be bent to conform to the joints. Unfortunately, even with these genuinely helpful devices there was often lasting deformity as well as immobility of the joint, a condition known as ankylosis.

In rare instances, excision (the surgical removal of part of the hip) was chosen by surgeons who believed that it offered a better alternative to amputation or traction, but this procedure carried a very high fatality rate. Of the sixty-six total hip excisions documented during the war, only six patients survived. And in none of the cases that involved the acetabulum (the socket part of the hip joint) did the patient survive the surgery.

Yet despite the staggering mortality rates associated with Civil War wounds, and surgery that was needed to treat them, the field of orthopedic medicine benefitted greatly in terms of new learning and the development of individual expertise.

Surgeons and physicians were desperately trying to save life and limb. It is undoubtedly true that in no other way could so many surgeons have gained so much experience and understanding of orthopedic injuries, and this carried over to the care of civilian patients in the post-war years. Equally important, innovations developed by American field surgeons, North and South, spread to European medical circles.

Surgeon teaching and training also improved significantly during the Civil War. In 1861 Lewis A. Sayre became the nation's first professor of orthopedic surgery, at Bellevue Medical College in New York City. He became widely known for using casts to treat spinal disorders, a technique which would later influence modern treatments for scoliosis.

Hospital for Special Surgery Is Founded

An important institution also came into being during the war years. In 1863, Dr. James Knight founded what is now the Hospital for Special Surgery, the U.S. first hospital to specialize in orthopedics. Knight's medical experience had come not in the army but through his work with a charitable organization called the New York Association for Improving the Condition of the Poor.

His chief focus was "the construction of appliances for the restoration of impaired powers of locomotion in children laboring under deformities both congenital and [those resulting from] infantile paralysis." It was this concern rather than Knight's actual accomplishments—unfortunately, most of his "appliances" turned out to be not very effective—that earned him a place in orthopedic history. That, plus the hospital he founded, which remains one of the foremost orthopedic hospitals in the country.

Many surgeons who had gained experience treating bone injuries during the war often went on to direct new orthopedic hospitals that opened after the war ended, and the practice of orthopedic surgery began to be recognized as a true specialty.

The American Orthopaedic Association was formed in 1887, becoming the first nationally organized group of orthopedic surgeons, and two years later the Association began to publish the proceedings of its meetings in *Transactions of the American Orthopaedic Association*, the original name of today's *Journal of Bone and Joint Surgery*.

These wartime and post-war advances in the *profession* of orthopedic medicine, along with increased sanitation and hygiene in the surgical arena and more effective treatment of infections, would continue to shape the practice of orthopedic surgery.

In short, the American Civil War was both a laboratory and a catalyst for future innovations, but the next great advances toward safe and effective hip surgery would not involve battlefield injuries, nor would they take place in the U.S.

Early Hip Surgery

Battle wounds and other trauma, of course, were not the only causes of serious hip problems. This is due to the nature of the hip itself.

The hip joint consists of two bones: the femur, or thigh, and the acetabulum, a kind of socket in the hipbone into which the femur extends.

The upper end of the femur is wider than the rest of the bone, forming a kind of ball that rotates smoothly—at least in healthy persons—within the joint. In fact, the hip is usually described as a ball-and-socket joint.

Over time, however, one or both bones can grind down, develop spurs or other deformities due to disease, or even break, although fractures of the acetabulum are comparatively rare. Because the hip joint must bear the body's weight, any significant deterioration of either bone can interfere with the joint's normal movement, causing severe pain that typically only worsens over time. Eventually, even the slightest movement can be excruciating.

Some skeletal problems are present at birth or develop at an early age. In the era before modern anti-bacterial drugs—sulfa would not be introduced until the 1930s and penicillin would not come into wide use until World War II—children and young adults in particular often were victims of acute joint infections that spread to vital organs. This meant that diseases of the joint were not only crippling—they could be fatal.

Among older adults, a common ailment was arthritis of the hip, or osteoarthritis, a condition which for many was manageable but which caused severe pain in others. Aside from opiates, the only relief in some cases was amputation, and as early as the eighteenth-century surgeons in America and Europe were experimenting with this procedure. But even as a last resort, this was not a satisfactory solution, and many surgeons continued to search for alternative treatments.

That search for a safe and more effective treatment would take decades, and the history of that search can have the appearance of a series of biographies—of physicians and surgeons, of inventors and technicians, and also of entrepreneurs and manufacturers.

A few of these individuals would gain renowned for their achievements, garnering honors and even knighthoods, but modern orthopedic surgery came about as the end result of many trials and many errors. The errors are forgivable: desperate situations can call for desperate measures, and several pioneers deserve special mention.

One early innovator was Henry Park of The Royal Infirmary in Liverpool, England. He had been appointed surgeon there 1767, and he practiced excision of the joint, a procedure in which part of the bone was removed and the remaining bone tissue was fused, and he became a strong advocate for its use as an alternative to amputation. But excision was presented greater difficulties for surgeons than amputation, and it was never widely accepted.

Another English surgeon, Anthony White of the Westminster Hospital in London, has been credited with performing the first excision arthroplasty in 1821. This did reduce pain, but the price was diminished stability.

Occasionally, the problem was not pain caused by movement within the hip, but by the fusion of the hip bones themselves, resulting in a rigid joint. This required an entirely different approach, and in 1825, in Philadelphia, Pennsylvania, John Rhea Barton performed the first osteotomy on a fused hip joint.

Osteotomy involves surgically removing part of the bone and reshaping the remaining bone to create a better alignment. The initial results of Barton's technique were positive, but over time the joint would become rigid again, and subsequent surgeries produced mixed results. There was also a high mortality rate with the procedure, approximately 50%. And repeated surgeries meant a greater likelihood of infection and death.

The next step in treating problems of the hip joint was the surgical placement of material into the joint itself, between the femur and the hip socket, a procedure called interposition.

Designed to reduce friction between the bones, the first known use of this technique was in 1860, by Auguste Stanislas Verneuil in Paris, who inserted neighboring soft tissue into the joint, but there was little interest in this procedure until Frenchman Léopold Ollier wrote about his own interposition of adipose tissue (basically body fat) into hip joints in the 1880s. Because he did not affix the tissue directly to the femur, his technique was only a half-step and never completely effective.

Shortly thereafter, in Breslau, Germany, Vitezlav Chlumsky experimented with a variety of interposed materials, including "muscle, celluloid, silver plates, rubber struts, magnesium, zinc, glass, Pyrex, decalcified bones, wax and celluloid." Again, none of these proved satisfactory, but Chlumsky was ahead of his time in another important respect: unlike most of his contemporaries, he would first try each material on animals before using it in humans.

Chlumsky's list of materials appears strange today but finding the right material for hip interpositions would remain a major goal of hip surgery a hundred years later.

The transition from simply inserting material into a joint to developing a prosthetic hip implant was led by Themistocles Glück in Germany in 1890. Glück used a ball and socket joint made out of ivory, which was fixed to the bone with nickel-plated screws. He also pioneered using bone cement. But despite these genuine advances, none of his implants was successful, possibly due to infections that had existed prior to surgery.

After the turn of the century, Robert Jones of Britain experimented with a novel technique: *covering* reconstructed femoral heads with gold foil. The procedure seemed to work well, and the patient "still retained effective motion at the joint" twenty-one years later. Deeply committed to advancing the treatment of fractures, Jones became a prominent figure in British orthopedics: in addition to his surgical accomplishments, he was instrumental in the founding of the British Orthopaedic Society in 1894, and in World War I he served as Inspector of Military Orthopedics, a position that enabled him to influence the care and treatment of soldiers suffering severe bone injuries.

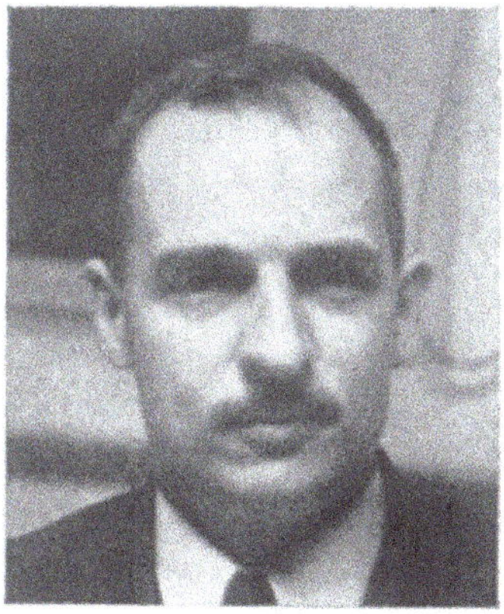 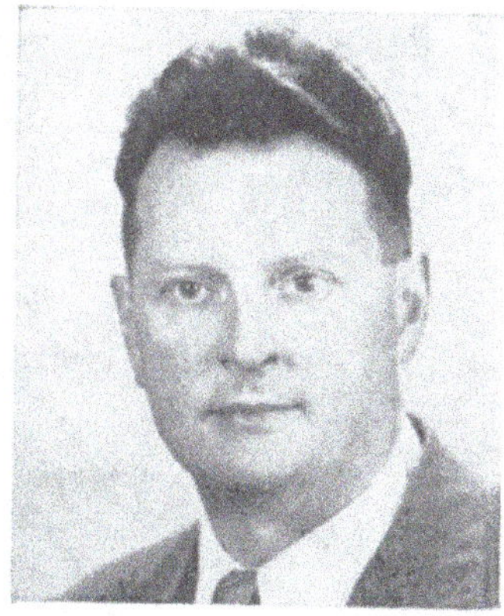

Robert and Jean Judet
Courtesy of Postgraduate Medical Journal; BMJ Journals

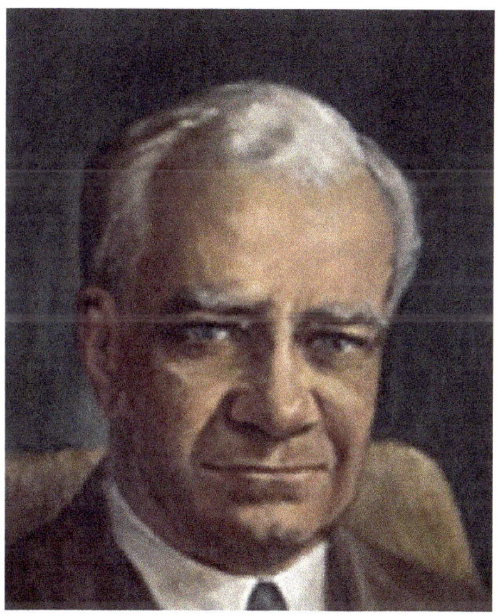

Marius Nygaard Smith-Petersen
Source: Cloudfront.net

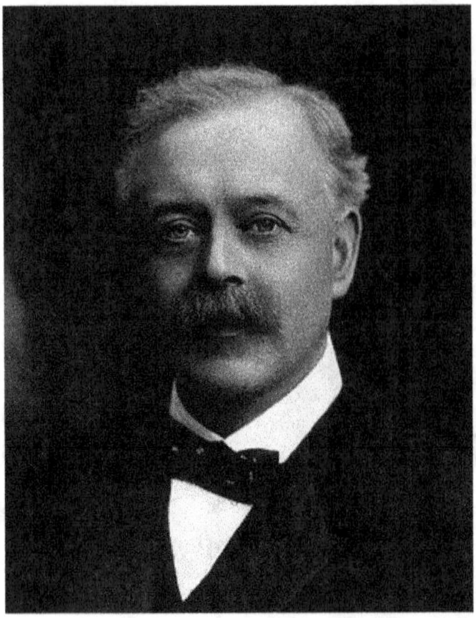

Sir Robert Jones / Source: Wikipedia.org

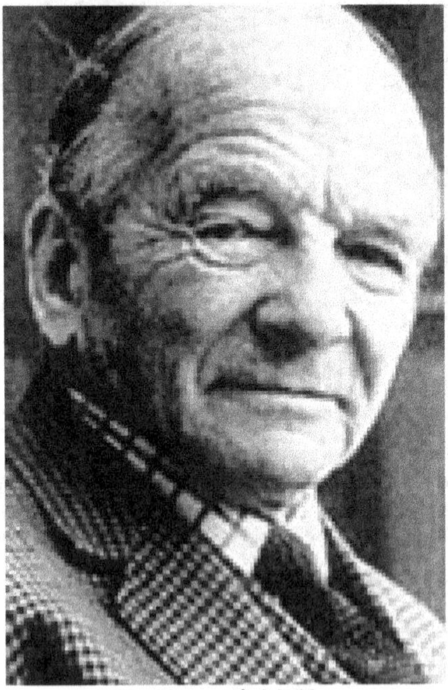

Dr. Kenneth McKee
Source: Joint Implant Surgery and Research Foundation

In the years before and immediately after WWI, three other surgical techniques were tried. One was the use of various natural materials in osteotomies, procedures in which the hip bone is cut, reshaped, or partially removed. The second was known as arthrodesis, the cutting away of part of the joint and then fixing the joint to prevent motion. The third procedure was the removal of the top end of the femur and the repositioning of the remaining femur upward into the hip socket to form a makeshift joint.

All were radical, high-risk operations with highly questionable results: each procedure inevitably resulted in a loss of mobility or stability, if not both, and none actually relieved pain, which usually had been the major reason for the procedure in the first place. Even worse, some patients were unable to walk at all afterwards.

Much better results were achieved in Boston in the 1920s when Norwegian-born Dr. Marius Smith-Petersen began to use synthetic materials in a variation of the then standard interposition procedure.

His approach was to place a cup-like glass mold between the femoral head (the top of the thigh bone) and the acetabulum to prevent the femoral bone itself from moving directly against the hip socket. This, he believed, would promote the growth of a smooth membrane around the glass and help the body heal itself. The idea was not guesswork on his part: Smith-Petersen had noticed the growth of such a membrane in an unrelated surgery.

Glass, however, proved to be too fragile—several molds broke—and he subsequently turned to other materials, including celluloid, Pyrex, and steel. It began to appear that nothing would work satisfactorily. Then in 1937, acting on a suggestion from his dentist, Smith-Petersen tried Vitallium, a trademarked chrome-cobalt alloy that was beginning to be used in dentistry.

The results were good if not spectacular—Smith-Petersen eventually achieved a 62.5% success rate—and his prosthesis became a popular option for patients with diseased acetabulums. He implanted some 500 Vitallium molds in all, but his procedure would not make its way to England until after World War II. By then, other researchers were looking at an even more promising technique.

Unexpected Breakthrough: The First Hip Replacement

Throughout the first decades of the twentieth century, orthopedic surgery still mainly focused on the femoral half of the hip joint, and various materials were tried in prostheses that replaced the femoral head, the top of the thigh that fits into the hip joint. But even if the right material could be found, this technique provided only a partial hip replacement (hemi-arthroplasty), and for many patients this meant only a partial solution.

An unexpected breakthrough came in 1938 when Philip Wiles performed the first total hip replacement at the Middlesex Hospital in London.

His femoral prosthesis was stainless steel and was held in place by a side plate secured by screws and bolts. It was a bold idea, but the procedure was not completely successful: of the six young patients who underwent the operation, all of them suffering from rheumatoid arthritis, only one could walk without pain thirteen years later. Still, it was a significant milestone.

Whether Wiles might have improved upon these initial results will never be known. Before he could follow up and refine his procedure, World War II intervened and the emphasis in orthopedics abruptly shifted, again, from birth defects and diseases to battlefield wounds.

During the war, it was mainly American surgeons who took the next steps. Physicians Austin Moore and Harold R. Bohlman, at John Hopkins Hospital in 1943, tried replacing the femoral head with a metal prosthesis fixed in place by a plate screwed to the outside of the femur in much the same manner that Wiles had developed. This side-plate fixation technique soon gave way to a better one in which one end of a metal rod (the stem) was inserted down into hollow core of the femur. This method gained wide acceptance, and in the early 1950s Moore refined his prosthesis by placing perforations in the stem to allow bone in-growth that aided in firmly fixing the device inside the femoral canal.

Working independently of Moore, Dr. Frederick R. Thompson of New York developed a similar prosthesis but with a femoral head made from a chrome-cobalt alloy. Like Moore's procedure, it dealt with only half of the joint, the femur, but their respective devices were key steps in developing methods and materials that would later be used in total hip arthroplasty.

In the years immediately following the war, another American, Edward Haboush, did attempt a total hip replacement, using Vitallium and an acrylic cement, but with poor results. The failure of his procedure has usually been attributed to his using the cement to glue the prosthesis to the bone rather than as a grout surrounding the stem to seal it within the bone canal.

More successful were two French brothers, Robert and Jean Judet, whose efforts attracted considerable interest. In 1946 they implanted a femoral prosthesis made from acrylic, a kind of plastic. Even though the device showed signs of wear almost immediately and was therefore not really suitable as an arthroplasty material, the design itself was adopted by others who would refine it and fabricate prostheses from a chrome-cobalt alloy.

The exchange of information about new various, both through journals and seminars, was critical to further advances, and throughout the 1950s orthopedic research continued to build on the methods and materials pioneered by Smith-Petersen, Moore and Bohlman, the Judet brothers, and, most importantly, Wiles.

In fact, it was Wiles' work in particular that shifted the focus back across the Atlantic to Britain, thanks in part to his textbook *Essentials of Orthopaedics*, first published in 1949. And the next significant step would be taken by a surgeon who had been one of Wiles' students.

Prior to World War II, Dr. Kenneth McKee had studied hip arthroplasty and had even made models of hip prostheses, but he had not yet experimented with any of them when, as with Wiles, military service interrupted his research. However, after the war McKee returned to the Norfolk and Norwich Hospital in England and essentially picked up where Wiles had left off.

Unlike other researchers, McKee worked mostly alone, except for collaborations with John Watson-Farrar, an orthopaedics colleague. And while others focused on improving femur-only implants, McKee was convinced that *total* hip replacement was the answer, especially when the hip socket itself was diseased. This meant making a prosthesis for the acetabulum in addition to one for the femoral head.

Initially using stainless steel for both, McKee attached the hip socket prosthesis with screws and inserted the femoral component (a stem with a ball at the top that fit into the socket) directly into the femur's shaft, basically following Thompson's design and using a plate and screws on the outside of the bone. In 1953 he began using Vinertia, an alloy of chrome and cobalt, but by the end of the decade his failure rate was still high—46%. The problem was prosthetic loosening: the prosthesis would not keep a firm fit.

McKee was on the right track, but his methods would soon be supplanted by an even better procedure, one developed by a fellow countryman.

CHAPTER TWO: JOINT REPLACEMENT

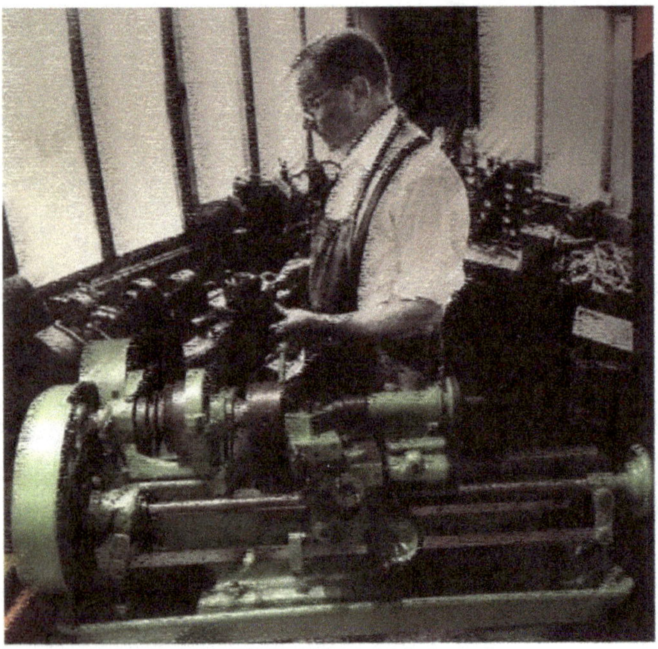

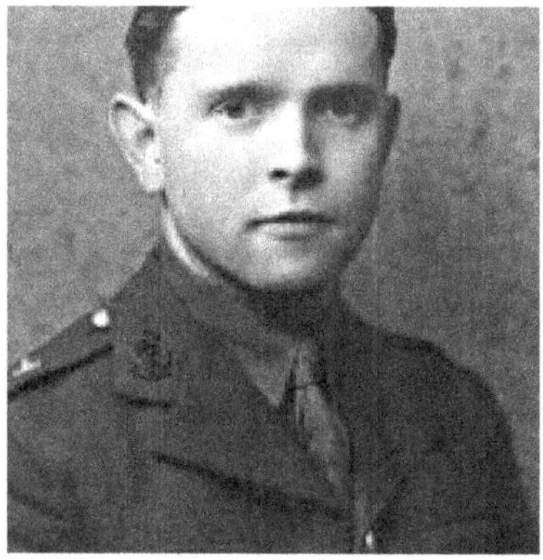

John Charnley is the father of modern orthopedic surgery. He showed how opening the human body, with proper technique, excising, sewing, nailing, implanting supremely well engineered instrumentation and implants, could fix hips, knees, shoulders, ankles, wrists, fingers, toes and the entire panoply of spinal trauma and disease—routinely.

It would take a little known engineer, Seth Greenwald, to bring scalability to Charnley's breakthrough. More about Dr. Greenwald later.

As can be said of most pioneers of consequence, Charnley was also complicated—at once a visionary and a relic. He laid the foundation for an entire branch of medicine and inspired legions of surgeons and engineers over the ensuing five decades.

He, however, defined this emerging branch in terms of pre-World War II surgical medicine (no antibiotics in surgery, for example).

Brilliant, flawed and compelling—here is the complicated story of Sir John Charnley.

From Dentistry to Orthopedics

John Charnley was born 1911 in Bury, England, a town of 55,000 people which dates back to the Roman era. He'd initially intended go into dentistry. His father operated a chemist shop where he also performed dentistry in a back room—but the headmaster at Charnley's school convinced him to choose medicine as a career instead.

At the age of eighteen, Charnley was accepted by the University of Manchester to study medicine, and while there he would have been exposed to lectures by Harry Platt, one of the leading British orthopedic surgeons of the time. Charnley graduated in 1935 and was awarded a fellowship from the Royal College of Surgeons of England in his first year as a physician.

Four years later, Charnley returned to Manchester where he simultaneously held two posts: resident casualty officer at the Manchester Royal Infirmary and assistant resident surgical officer. These duties kept him extremely busy, but the work gave him valuable surgical experience and brought him into contact with orthopedic injuries for the first time. It so happened that the orthopedic unit was supervised by none other than Platt himself, who was assisted by Henry Osmond-Clarke. Both men were influential in guiding Charnley towards specializing in orthopedics and orthopedic surgery, but there may have been an additional factor in his decision, an incident that had occurred when Charnley was still a student.

He was a member of the university's mountaineering club, and during a climbing trip a fellow student took a bad fall and fractured his thigh bone. The injury was severe, but the climbers could not leave the top of the climb due to darkness. Charnley applied a splint to the leg, but during the night the injured student succumbed to shock. To what degree this tragedy affected Charnley's career choice is not known, but such an event undoubtedly would have had an impact on any young doctor.

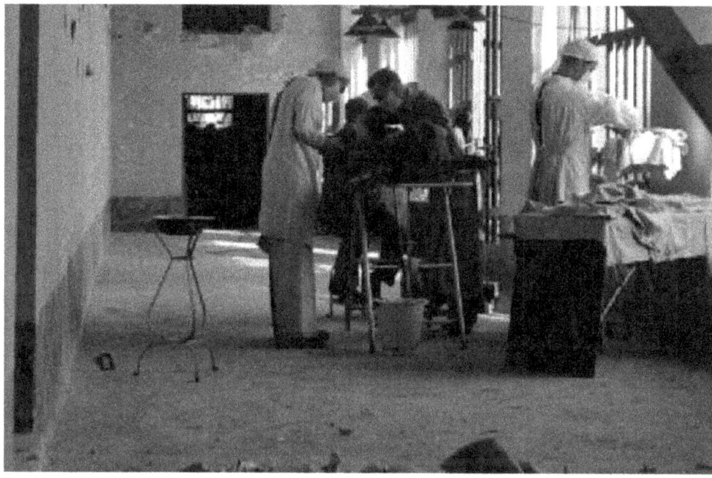

British surgeons at work during World War II

For Charnley the Second World War was a pivotal experience. Joining the Royal Army Medical Corps in May 1940, he spent the majority of his military service in Cairo, Egypt, where he came to the attention of St. John Dudley Buxton. Buxton's duties included the organization of military orthopedic centers in the Middle East, and he soon noticed Charnley's abilities, assigning him a variety of responsibilities, one of which was to have important consequences.

Among his duties was supervision of a machine shop, where Charnley was responsible for manufacturing appliances and surgical instruments for one of the Cairo centers. His work there, together with his natural mechanical skills, added to his knowledge of metalworking, an expertise that would be of enormous benefit later. Buxton was also probably responsible for Charnley's being invited to join, as an associate member, the British Orthopaedic Association in 1943. Charnley remained in Cairo from the fall of 1941 to May 1944, when he was sent back to England to serve as orthopedic surgeon at the military hospital in Shaftesbury, England.

Following his discharge from military service in 1946, Charnley returned to Manchester to resume work with Platt, who soon sent him to one of the peripheral country orthopedic hospitals. It was an assignment that exposed Charnley to elective orthopedic surgery.

For the first time he was treating patients afflicted with bone and joint tuberculosis, with poliomyelitis, or with other diseases. All were problems for which corrective surgery appeared appropriate.

After six months he returned to Manchester, and in 1947, following Harry Platt's retirement, Charnley was named Consultant Orthopaedic Surgeon at the Manchester Royal Infirmary and visiting orthopedic surgeon at Wrightington Hospital near Wigan, in northwest England.

It was the latter appointment that would turn out to be central to Charnley's future research.

The Idea of a Total Hip Replacement Takes Root

By 1951, many orthopedic surgeons, with the notable exception of McKee, were beginning to believe that total hip replacement would never be a viable surgical option. Charnley himself had given serious thought to the problems that would be encountered in such surgery—in fact, he claimed to have even designed a hip arthroplasty as early as 1946 but had abandoned the procedure after a preliminary trial proved unsuccessful—and he likewise had become pessimistic about whether total hip replacement was feasible.

Charnley did not completely stop thinking about hip arthroplasty, especially for patients with osteoarthritis in both hip joints and those suffering from rheumatoid arthritis, an inflammation of the membrane that protects the joints. He also became intrigued when a patient who had received a Judet acrylic prosthesis complained that his hip would squeak when he leaned forward and that the noise was so pronounced that his wife would leave the room. It was not an isolated incident either: Charnley was aware of other patients with Judet hips that exhibited the same phenomenon, typically about two years after surgery, although the squeaking would eventually disappear.

Charnley believed the squeaking was caused by friction between the femoral prosthesis and the hip socket and that the underlying problem was a lack of lubrication inside the joint. The squeaking stopped, he thought, only because of loosening of the prosthesis in the socket, not because of improved lubrication. This insight sent him on a search for a way to lubricate the artificial joint or, failing that, to find a material that would lessen resistance and friction and also be suitable for insertion in human bodies.

Charnley Rejects Lubricating the Hip, Narrows the Problem

After an exhaustive study of the science of lubrication—both biological and mechanical—Charnley concluded there simply was no way to introduce a lubricant into the joint.

That left just two options: either the prosthesis itself would need a permanent coating, such as that naturally produced by the body in healthy joints, or the material from which the prostheses was fabricated would have to be of a type that produced minimal friction.

Every solid has a "coefficient of friction"—the higher the coefficient number, the greater the friction—and the coefficient of friction for normal joint cartilage is, to quote Charnley's own words, "phenomenally low." In his search for such a "slippery substance," Charnley made contact with Henry Crossley, the owner of Henry Crossley Limited, a company that was then looking into new uses for a new product. The product's chemical name was polytetrafluorethylene, or PTFE, but it would become better known by its trade name, Teflon.

Although the effects of this product on the human body were unknown at the time, the material was believed to be inert in the human body, and its low surface friction characteristics made it appear to be the ideal material for Charnley's purposes. Indeed, the notion of introducing a "slippery surface" (in this case, Teflon) marked a key advance over McKee's work at Norwich; because there was no longer a need for continued lubrication, low-friction arthroplasty was now feasible.

Charnley Goes Single-Cup and Excises the Femoral Head

At some point between 1956 and 1958, Charnley began experimenting with the material in his own hip arthroplasty cases. At first, he used a "double-cup" technique, in which PTFE was applied to the acetabulum, forming a kind of thin cup, while a second cup coated with the material covered the femoral head.

The aim was to reproduce the kind of coatings found naturally in the joint. While the procedure produced good results in pain relief and movement, Charnley realized that the femoral cup would inhibit blood supply to the bone, and he decided to try a different approach, using only one cup. He optimistically hinted at such a modification in a 1959 lecture delivered to a division of the British Medical Association, saying it was "probable" that a prosthetic "femoral prosthesis, articulating with a PTFE socket" would work better than his original double-cup design.

This next step required the removal of the femoral head by excision and replacing it with a prosthesis of the type used by Moore but keeping the acetabulum PTFE cup Charnley had developed.

His engineering colleagues also convinced him to make the diameter of the femoral ball as small as possible to further reduce friction and to allow for a thicker acetabulum cup. This would help prevent slippage of the cup within the hip socket. The final result was a femoral prosthesis with a ball approximately half the diameter of Moore's device. Other surgeons would question the wisdom of this final change, but Charnley would remain steadfast in his belief that his approach was the correct one.

Acrylic Dental Cement

He also decided to add acrylic dental cement to fix the femoral device. Not that using cement to fix an implant to bone was a new idea. Some 70 years earlier, Gluck had tried this, using a variety of materials including an alloy of copper and mercury, "plaster of Paris, and stone putty (rosin with pumice stone or gypsum)." And as recently as 1953, Haboush had used dental acrylic cement to affix the two parts of his prosthesis. But Charnley would use the cement not as adhesive, but as grout to make a better in-bone fit.

Now all Charnley had to do was make the devices and surgically implant them. Because he knew exactly what he wanted, he initially fabricated them in his attic workshop. Charnley felt confident that he had found the formula for total hip replacement.

Charles F. Thackray Ltd and Harry Craven Join Charnley

The exact date that Charnley performed his first total hip replacement using PTFE—he always called it "low-friction arthroplasty"—and the name of the first patient who received the new prosthesis are not known. Part of the confusion is due to Charnley's own later, but inconsistent, accounts, but it was probably in 1956. Two years later he hired a technician, Harry Craven, to take over the actual fabricating process, although if a piece needed modification Charnley would typically make the changes himself. Only when both men were satisfied with the design would the prototype be sent to Charles F. Thackray Ltd., in Leeds for manufacture. The relationship with Thackray was long-standing, having begun in 1947 when Thackray replaced Charnley's previous supplier of "hip fracture devices." The Thackray company itself had started out as a retail pharmacy but had been deeply involved in the manufacture of surgical equipment since the end of World War I.

Charnley opened a special bio-mechanical workshop in 1961, and a year later he installed a wear testing machine to evaluate the characteristics and suitability of various materials, including PTFE, for implants. For a while, everything went well—Charnley performed approximately 300 apparently successful hip replacements using PTFE cups—but a major problem began to appear. The same year that he began testing material in his new workshop, Charnley discovered that particles that had worn off the acetabular cup were

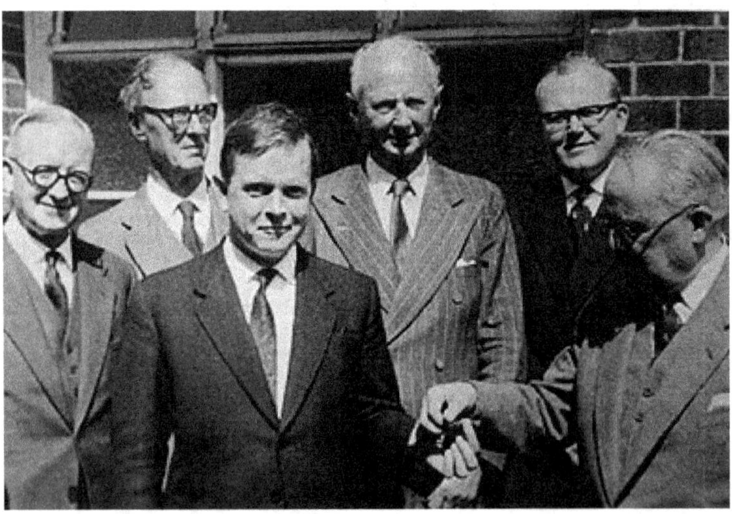

Young Dr. Charnley Received the keys to his lab 1961.

causing some "adverse tissue reactions" in patients over the three-year period that PTFE had been used. Charnley had even detected some wear in the cups after the first year, but he had assumed this was a normal "bedding-in" process and would subside in time. In fact, the wear continued, tripling after three years. Moreover, while the wearing itself was troubling enough, the particles were causing material masses to form around the joint and were destroying the bone itself.

Deeply concerned, Charnley injected PTFE particles into his own thigh to determine once and for all whether the product itself was the cause. It was. When the mass in his leg increased in size over a nine-month period, he knew that the material could no longer be safely used and that the cups already implanted had to be removed. Patients were notified, and he performed each revision surgery himself. It was a setback that made Charnley an extremely cautious man.

Craven Tests a New Plastic

At about the same time, Craven was quietly testing a sample of a new plastic that had been developed in Germany to make plastic gears and which was being used locally in Lancashire textile machinery. The material was "ultra-high molecular weight polyethylene," UHMWPE for short.

Craven had showed the sample to Charnley, who had told Craven he was wasting his time. Fortunately, Craven ignored Charnley's advice and began testing a sample.

The results were immediate and striking after three weeks of continuous testing, the new plastic still did not show as much wear as PTFE had exhibited in only twenty-four hours.

Charnley was now interested, but because of his experience with Teflon he again experimented on himself by placing small samples in his own thigh. The new product appeared to be inert in humans, but Charnley was taking no chances.

After six months, when there were still no discernible effects from the sample in his thigh, and after some further testing in the workshop he concluded that HMWP was indeed safe to use. Charnley performed the first arthroplasty using the new plastic in November 1962.

Although Charnley, ever cautious, did not immediately publish the results of his revised procedure, word spread of his success. Within a year, the demand for his devices had grown to the point that increased production of implant devices was needed. Craven had been making the cups in the biomechanical workshop as needed, but Charnley asked him to build a machine that would produce the parts faster.

He did, and the machine was later sold to Thackray. The femoral prosthesis was forged from stainless steel by a company in Sheffield, then taken to Thackray where it was machined to its final shape. Final polishing was then done at Wrightington.

Eureka! But Charnley Blocks Wide Distribution

Surgeons were naturally anxious to learn more about his breakthrough, but there was a hitch. Charnley himself had a strong working knowledge of physical mechanics—thanks largely to his army posting in Cairo—but he was doubtful as to whether other surgeons had the requisite understanding and skill. In his view, as reported in a 1959 lecture to a division of the British Medical Association, total hip replacement required "training in mechanical techniques which, though elementary in practical engineering, are as yet unknown in the training of a surgeon."

He was determined to rectify this oversight: only surgeons who visited the Center and agreed to undergo at least two and a half days of training (to learn Charnley's specific procedures) were permitted to purchase the devices from Thackray. Even then, not all surgeons who wanted to attend were accepted by Charnley.

This sharply limited Thackray's profits, and it also created resentment among surgeons who felt they should be allowed to purchase the prosthesis based on their reputation alone. By 1968 Thackray was needing more sales if it was going to continue manufacturing the devices, and Charnley agreed to no longer require that surgeons have his personal approval before training at the Center.

But he still insisted that any surgeon who wished to purchase his devices from Thackray first had to attend at least a two-day training session at Wrightington. Even this final restriction would be lifted a few years later, thereafter, allowing anyone to purchase a prosthesis from Thackray.

Charnley's cautious approach was evident in other respects as well. One was his decision to offer his arthroplasty only to elderly patients—those older than sixty-eight years of age—who had severe disabilities. His philosophy in this regard put him at odds with

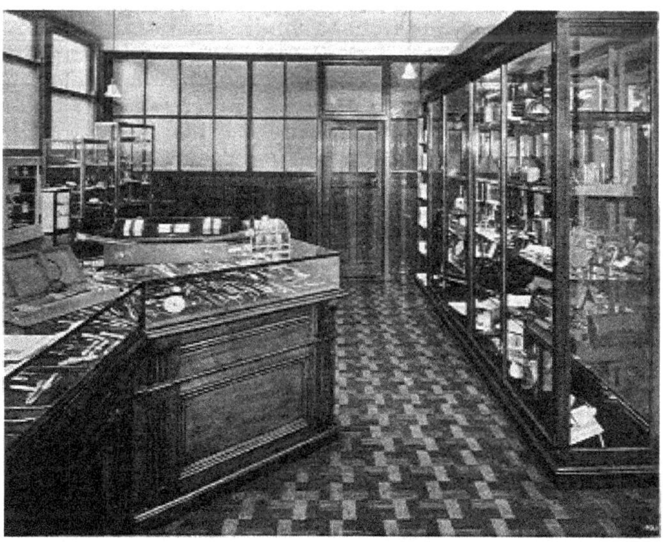

21. Thackray's showroom at Park Street, known as the front shop, where surgeons could call in person to buy instruments.

Thackray's showroom at Park Street in London circa:

prevailing attitude of American surgeons, who believed that hip replacement should be primarily used for younger patients and those who could be expected to lead a more active life after surgery. But even with these age and disability restrictions, Charnley had no shortage of patients. By 1967, upwards of 700 total hip replacements were being performed every year at Wrightington.

Charnley Meets Seth Greenwald

Although his accomplishments had become widely known, Charnley declined to publish his research until he was certain that the long-term results were positive—he was not about to risk a repeat of the Teflon experience. When he finally did publish, ten years after his first use of HMWP, he was able to report that 90% of his patients had no pain whatsoever after surgery, with the remaining patients indicating only slight or intermittent pain. Of those patients who had been able to walk only a limited distance with the aid of crutches or canes before the surgery, over 80% claimed to be able to walk, unaided, an unlimited distance afterwards.

Despite Charnley's reluctance to allow sales of his prostheses to surgeons unfamiliar with his procedure, he gladly shared information about his procedure—once he was satisfied there were no hidden problems.

In the early fall of 1968, John Charnley, then 57 years old was on his way into the Oxford University to give yet another talk. Charnley who would eventually be knighted for his accomplishment, was standing on the shoulders of several giants of orthopedic surgery—both surgical and commercial—notably, Friedrich Pauwels (1885-1980) who laid down basic concepts of hip biomechanics in the early 1900s, the German company Hoechst whose Ultra High Molecular Weight (UHMWP) polymer was the final puzzle piece for Charnley and the Copenhagen company Kaler and Jansen and their acrylic bone cement which Charnley would always refer to as the 'grout' interface between metal and bone.

Little did Charnley know, as he made the 246 mile trip to London that day that he was about to meet a student, an aeronautical engineer named Seth Greenwald, who would change orthopedics as much, probably more, than he did.

Indeed, this MIT and Columbia university grad, who was at Oxford University to earn his doctorate, would wind up turning the entire musculoskeletal industry away from the then prevailing method of designing, testing, approving and ultimately, commercializing orthopedic and spinal implants and instruments.

That student would also challenge, to Charnley's chagrin, the prevailing wisdom that the human hip was a ball and socket joint.

Greenwald spent five years in aerospace engineering before leaving to pursue a doctoral degree at Oxford University in England. In 1968, his professor and advisor, Dr. Robert Duthie, the Nuffield Professor of Orthopedics at Oxford said to Greenwald, "We have this chap Charnley coming. He's doing this experimental surgery." And Duthie, who actually wasn't sure Charnley's surgery would ever catch on, asked Greenwald to put together a companion talk about biomechanics of the hip.

Which Greenwald did. His lab work was published in the journal *Nature*, titled: *Incongruent Surfaces in the Human Hip*.

To measure the articulating surfaces of the hip joint, Greenwald invented a three-legged gauge which measured the curvature of both the femoral head and the acetabulum surfaces of the hip joint. He used 53 cadaver hips of widely varying ages to gather data. He calculated the radius of curvature at four points which were equidistant from each other along an equatorial circle. The data clearly showed that there were substantial differences in curvature from point to point on both the acetabular and the femoral head.

The joint surfaces, Greenwald proved, were not spherical and could not be congruent. Furthermore, said Greenwald, because the hip joint is incongruent, the site and size of the actual contact areas will depend on the position of the joint and the magnitude and direction of the applied load.

Bottom line, the human hip did not articulate as a ball and socket joint!

By inference, then, a ball and socket prosthesis could well alter the direction and strength of biomechanical forces in the hip, the adjoining spine, the knee...essentially radiating entirely new forces throughout the musculoskeletal system.

Charnley, who based his hip replacement design on the premise that the hip was a ball and socket joint, gave his presentation at the Imperial College of London first. Greenwald spoke next. A few days later, Charnley sent a sharply critical note telling Greenwald he was absolutely wrong and furthermore, after performing hundreds of hip surgeries he knew, as any idiot could also tell, that human hips were balls and sockets.

Greenwald would later take his aeronautical engineering approach as well as the Oxford style of debate and didactic education to, first, Cleveland Clinic, Charity Hospital, then to Mueller and the nascent AO Foundation and, finally, to the FDA where he served as one of the first Orthopedic Panel chairmen.

Charnley, Müller and the AO

After his *Nature* paper in 1968 and the back and forth with John Charnley, Greenwald's star was rising. Henry Mankin, M.D., who'd recently left New York's Hospital for Joint Disease (now better known as the NYU Langone Orthopedic Hospital, arguably the preeminent orthopedic academic center in the world) for Harvard where he accepted the Edith M. Ashley Professorship of Orthopedic Surgery, was a growing fan. C. McCollister Evarits, one of Oxford University Robert Duthie's protégée's, was now Chief of Orthopedics at the Cleveland Clinic and would become instrumental in getting Greenwald to Cleveland.

In 1974, Maurice Edmond Müller M.D., professor at the University of Bern and head of orthopedic surgery at the Inselspital in Bern asked Greenwald to come to Switzerland and design a proper orthopedic laboratory.

Müller, who co-founded the AO Foundation (Arbeitsgemeinschaft für Osteosynthesefragen) had visited Charnley's Wrightington lab many times during the 1960s. In 1967, one year before Charnley's fateful meeting with Greenwald, Müller started his own large-scale production of Charnley's hip through Protek AG (which later merged with Sulzer Medica, and then spun off as Centerpulse and, finally, acquired by Warsaw, Indiana based Zimmer, Inc.).

Charnley agreed to lend his name to the Protek manufactured implant and the Charnley-Müller prosthesis was born.

Then...Müller decided to make the prosthetic head bigger (30mm), increase the number of neck lengths and drop Charnley's osteotomy of the great trochanter in order to apply the femoral component.

Charnley was not happy. He retracted his support saying in a 1970 letter, "*...those manufacturers who in the past have made the Charnley-Müller with the 30 mm head should now drop my name. Müller attached my name to his prosthesis out of courtesy because we are close personal friends and because he was acknowledging my pioneer work...The situation has now changed in so far as my operation is certainly a more extensive mechanical procedure than his....*"

Greenwald spent two months in 1974 in Switzerland with Mueller, developing a plan for a first-of-its-kind orthopedic R&D lab—which meant creating:

- ✓ An electronics facility to develop and fabricate electro/mechanical surgical instruments.
- ✓ A machine shop for prototyping new surgical tools and implants.
- ✓ A histology lab to prepare biological and implant material for microscopic analysis.
- ✓ A tissue and biomaterials lab to study the failure modes of new biomaterials.
- ✓ An illustration and reproduction facility to create graphs, charts, exhibits.
- ✓ An animal surgical suite
- ✓ A film studio and gait laboratory to support educational and information dissemination.
- ✓ Animal facilities,
- ✓ A bio-mechanical and materials testing lab,
- ✓ Project research labs which visiting surgeons could use to carry out their personal research.

Greenwald also proposed that the Müller foundation integrate an educational program for visiting surgeons. Müller accepted it all and asked Greenwald to stay on as the lab's first director.

Greenwald deferred, returning to Cleveland, eventually, to put almost precisely the same plan he'd given Müller and start the Cleveland Research Institute... where the modern spinal implant industry would first take root.

In 2002, the International Society of Orthopaedic Surgery and Traumatology (SICOT) named Müller the "Orthopaedic Surgeon of the Century".

As for Charnley, over the years his antipathy for the Müller/Greenwald approach grew. In speeches and writing, he expressed his staunch skepticism of the AO techniques and principles maintaining that the best experimental model was inferior to an adequate clinical judgment.

Charnley also did not patent his original design, which led to the copying of his prosthesis by others, although he later did obtain patents on some instruments and other innovations.

When he realized that he could not keep others from using his name in connection with the copies, he asked that competing products carry both his name and that of the imitator, creating a hyphenated name, such as the Charnley-Müller prosthesis, an arrangement that Charnley had previously authorized. In fact, the Charnley-Müller device was different from Charnley's in two important details. The copy's femoral head was half again as large as Charnley's and was fabricated from chrome-cobalt instead.

Other manufacturers produced their own variations, again using Charnley's name. In response, Charnley attempted to copyright his name to prevent imitators from passing their prostheses off as Charnley-authorized products without his express approval.

Nonetheless, the Charnley-Müller prosthesis gained popularity in the U.S. because of its larger femoral head size, its material (chrome-cobalt), and the fact that the surgical procedure with this implant did not require the removal and reattachment of the greater trochanter section of the femur. Thackray later produced chrome-cobalt prostheses to compete with other manufacturers in the American market, but the product failed to perform as well as the competition and eventually was dropped. Charnley himself never used anything but stainless steel.

Surgeons also adopted another Wrightington innovation: conducting surgery inside a "sterile air tent." Charnley was unwilling to rely on antibiotics to deal with infection; he was determined to minimize the risk of infection in the first place. To accomplish this, he worked with F. Hugh Howorth (of Howorth Air Engineering) to create "an ultra-clean operating environment." Besides the enclosure itself, called a "greenhouse," they designed impermeable masks and gowns that were vented by a built-in air exhaust system. The overall effect was to reduce the postoperative infection rate from 9% to less than 1%.

Charnley officially retired in 1975 but continued to conduct research on, and write about, orthopedics. He had truly changed the world of orthopedic surgery, and for his many accomplishments, especially the hip replacement innovations he developed, he garnered numerous honors in Britain and would be knighted in 1977, five years before his death. By then his hip replacement procedure had indeed become "the gold standard" in orthopedic hip surgery.

Besides his direct contributions to orthopedic surgery, Charnley left still another legacy, one that was epitomized by his long, albeit troubled, relationship with Thackray. If total hip replacement was to be a safe and reliable surgical option, quality prostheses and other critical components were essential. In this regard, as with surgery itself, Charnley was a perfectionist.

In addition to a prosthetic femoral stem and acetabular cup, two other manufactured devices were needed: screws or nails to hold the cup in place, and tools to perform the procedure.

Moreover, any component that was to remain in the body had to be made of an inert material—it must neither react to surrounding body tissue nor induce a reaction that would cause the body to reject the implant. Fine polishing, the last step in the manufacturing process, ensured that the surface of the prosthesis was as smooth as possible.

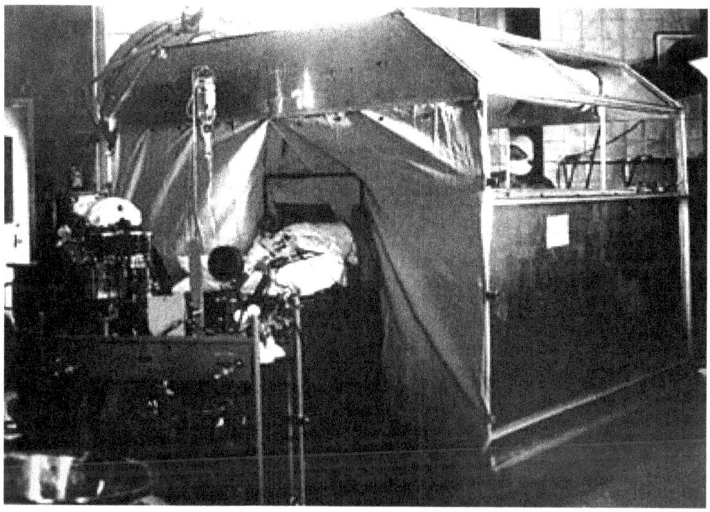

Sir John Charnley in his "sterile air tent" developed by F. Hugh Howorth.

Of course, none of these items was already on the shelf waiting to be ordered. Each device had to be designed and manufactured, usually by companies that had beginnings unrelated to surgery, let alone orthopedic implants. They were in a new field as well and would be called upon to manufacture products that met exacting quality standards. Thackray had once been a retail pharmacy, while other British companies had equally diverse origins. So, too, in the United States, where the first three American manufacturers started out as makers of customized splints.

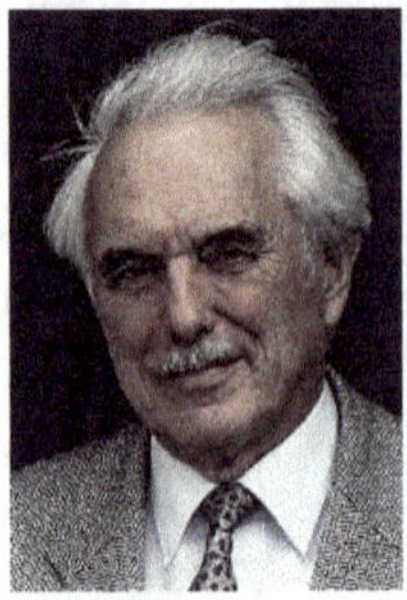

A Swiss surgeon and entrepreneur, Dr. Müller developed many internal fixation techniques to treat bone fractures and significantly advanced hip prostheses development. He has been honored with numerous awards including when the International Society of Orthopaedic Surgery and Traumatology (SICOT) named him the "Orthopedic Surgeon of the Century" at a congress in San Diego. Müller was also the patron who founded the Zentrum Paul Klee in Berne, Switzerland.

In 1958, Müller co-founded the Arbeitsgemeinschaft für Osteosynthesefragen. Inspired by the work of Belgian surgeon Robert Danis, Müller developed new tools and fixation implants for orthopedic surgery, marketed by Synthes Holding AG. In 1960 he became chair of the department of orthopedics and traumatology at the hospital of St. Gallen. From 1963 to 1980 he was professor at the University of Berne and head of orthopedic surgery at the Inselspital in Berne.

Profits from Müller's companies funded the Maurice E. Müller foundation and, over the years, other foundations which advanced orthopedic surgery education and research.

Henry Mankin

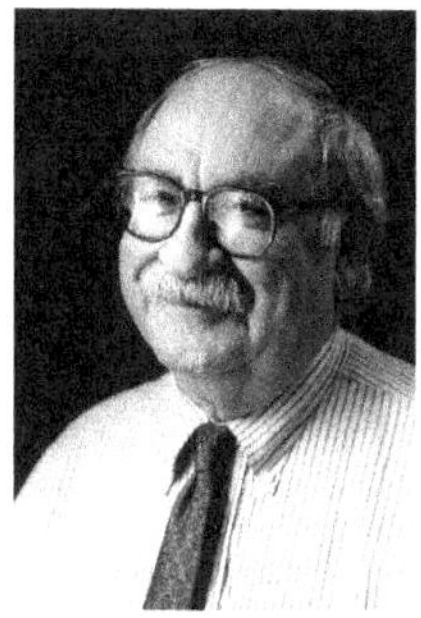

A Pittsburgh native, Dr. Mankin graduated from The School of Medicine at the University of Pittsburgh in the Class of 1953. In 1960, Dr. Mankin completed his orthopedic surgery residency at the Hospital for Joint Disease in New York, where he started his career as a professor and director of orthopedics, followed by time at Mt. Sinai Hospital before ultimately moving to Boston in 1972. A t Mass General, Dr. Mankin was Chief of Orthopedic Surgery from 1972 to 1996, as well as the Edith M Ashley Professor of Orthopedic Surgery at Harvard Medical School. Upon arrival to Mass General, he brought fellow orthopedic educators, including the late Drs. Richard Smith, Michael Ehrlich, and Robert Leffert.

Dr. Mankin wrote more than 600 publications and world-renowned lectures. Dr. Henry Mankin left an indelible mark on orthopedic surgery and the world in general.

CHAPTER THREE: THE PRACTICES OF SUPPLYING AND EDUCATING ORTHOPEDIC SURGEONS EMERGES IN WARSAW AND MEMPHIS

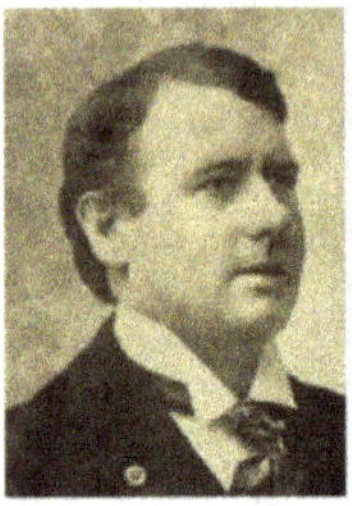

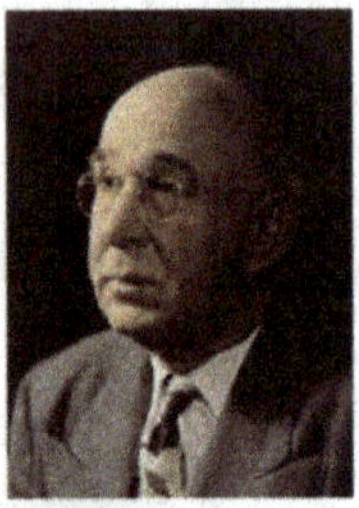

Revra DePuy (left) and Justin Zimmer (right).

City of Memphis Downtown circa 1910

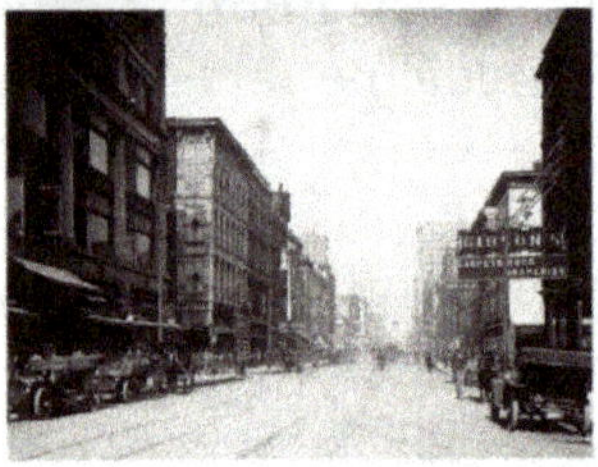

First Edition of Campbell's Operative Orthopaedics Textbook 1939

Dr. Willis Cohoon Campbell

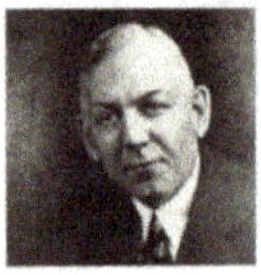

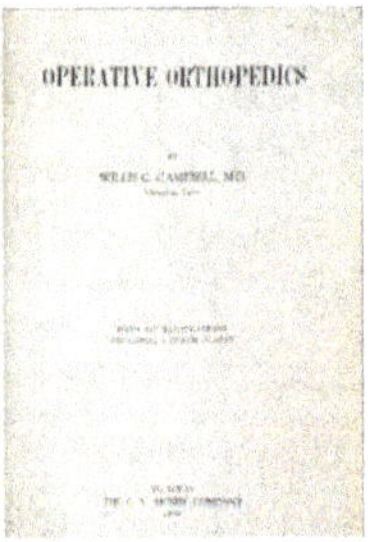

The business of orthopedics began as a splint, sling, neck collar and wound and fracture repair business—which, more formally, is called Trauma.

The basic technology of orthopedics in the first half of the 20th century was developed, literally, in early Egypt, around 3,000 B.C. These early trauma fixation tools were made of wood, and wood would remain the material of choice for millennia, although virtually any material strong enough to support an injured limb would work.

Because of their flat and relatively smooth surfaces, wooden barrel staves became very popular and were still being used in the U.S. in the late nineteenth century.

One man, Revra DePuy, is credited with launching, in the 19th century, the orthopedic supply business.

Revra DePuy

Revra DePuy was born in 1860 in Grand Rapids, Michigan. Although his family briefly moved to Canada when he was still a boy, young Revra's mother brought the family back to the Midwest after her husband died, settling in Marseilles, Illinois, about 80 miles southwest of Chicago.

When he was old enough, DePuy took on a variety of jobs, and one of them made a lasting impression. Working as a clerk in a local drug store, he became interested in medicine and chemicals, and he pursued this interest when he enrolled in the University of Toronto. There he received a degree in chemistry and upon graduation became a traveling pharmaceutical salesman, work that took him to Warsaw, Indiana, a small town in the north-central part of the state. The locale apparently appealed to him: when he later decided to open his own business, he chose Warsaw as his base. He already knew what he wanted to do.

DePuy was convinced that carefully designed splints would work far better than the wooden, often improvised ones routinely used by doctors of the time, and in 1895 DePuy Manufacturing became the first commercial orthopedic company in the United States. Its initial products were indeed fiber splints, and the Unites States Army became the company's best customer. The product line would soon include "slings, neck collars, and braces."

For a while, the business was headquartered in a Warsaw hotel, but in 1901 DePuy relocated to Niles, Michigan, just across the state line, enticed by incentives offered by leading citizens of that town. This move turned out to be temporary, however, because DePuy's products did not sell well in Michigan, and after only three years he moved the plant back to Warsaw.

A year after his return DePuy made an employment decision that would have significant consequences not only within the field of fracture appliances, but in an industry that did not yet even exist—the manufacturing of orthopedic implants. That decision was to hire twenty-year-old Justin O. Zimmer as his first sales representative.

The young man had been born on the family farm south of Warsaw, and he had later attended school to become a Western Union telegraph operator. He must not have enjoyed the work, however, because the same day he finished his telegraphy training he went to work as a DePuy splint salesman instead. Zimmer would stay with DePuy's company more than twenty years, the last five as sales manager, and when he did leave he would quickly demonstrate that he had learned the business well.

DePuy Manufacturing grew rapidly and by 1919 had sixteen full-time employees, including six salesmen who traveled the country as DePuy himself once had. When Revra DePuy died in 1921, his widow Winifred took over company operations. At that time, women heading any businesses, let alone a manufacturing business, were rare, but she did very well, managing the business and her marriage to Herschel Leiter in 1924.

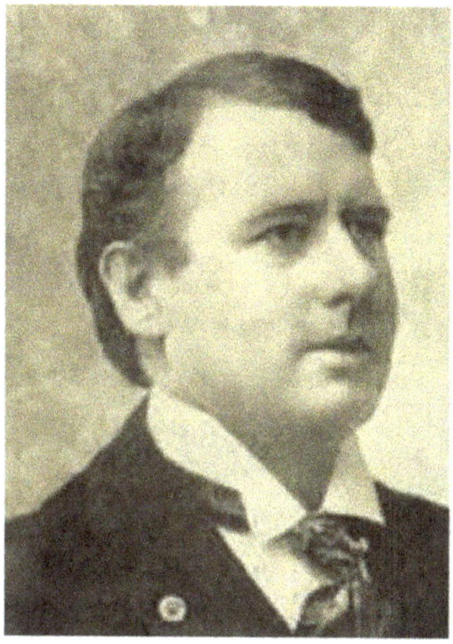 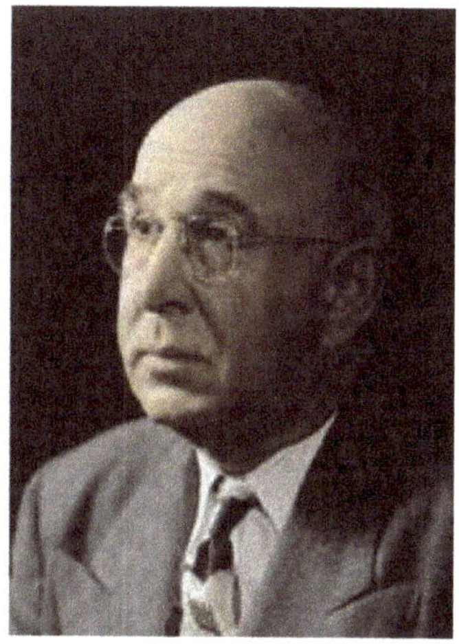

Revra DePuy (left) and Justin Zimmer (right).
Images courtesy of Medical Milestones by Symone Skrzycki

Justin Zimmer

When Justin Zimmer finally left DePuy in 1926, he was not just *changing* jobs. He left to set up his own splint-making business, and he persuaded some key DePuy employees to join him. One story has Zimmer, in the months before his departure, making copies of all of DePuy's products. This kind of move—learning the company business and then striking out on one's own in a similar enterprise—would be repeated many times in the industry over the next four decades, and the circumstances of his departure would become part of industry lore.

According to Zimmer, he had approached Winifred a year earlier with two proposals. He suggested adding aluminum splints to the company's product line, and he *asked* to buy an interest in the company. This was not the first time Zimmer had raised the partnership issue with her—he wanted to be more than an employee—but she dismissed both ideas out of hand. The Zimmer company history records his reaction: "I have had it," Mr. Zimmer told his wife and daughter that evening. "She said to me: 'You know, Justin, you are just small potatoes!'"

Rebuffed and certainly angry at being so casually dismissed, he was able to find two investors, William Felkner and William Rogers, willing to back him, and a year after Zimmer left DePuy the Zimmer Manufacturing Company set up shop in the basement of Zimmer's home in Warsaw. Assisting Zimmer were two former DePuy employees, J. J. Ettinger and Dr. C. F. Lytle, who helped create and market Zimmer's new aluminum splints and other orthopedic devices. Ettinger was the factory manager, while Lytle, a physician who had worked as a salesman at DePuy, worked alongside Zimmer. Zimmer also hired his former secretary at DePuy as office manager. Ettinger would later recall that local "experts" were convinced that there simply was not enough business for two splint manufacturing companies.

By the following May, Zimmer Manufacturing had fabricated enough products to be able to display samples of its new aluminum splints at that year's American Medical Association conference in Washington, D.C. The response was enthusiastic. Zimmer's product line was so popular that the company soon had to employ a nine-man sales network, and its catalog began advertising a total of fifty aluminum splints. In just seven months of operation, company sales surpassed those of DePuy, Justin Zimmer's former employer, for the entire previous year.

With demand for its products surging, the new firm soon outgrew its basement facilities and moved its operations to a building on North Detroit Street in Warsaw. It also developed additional product lines, including what it called "the fracture bed," a device that enabled hospital staff to change the bed sheeting without disturbing the patient. Profits were routinely plowed back into the business to purchase new equipment and further expand the size of the plant. In 1929, the same year the stock market collapsed, the company sold its first splints overseas, to a Scottish surgeon. This was no fluke: it was the beginning of a trend. Even during the harshest days of the Great Depression, Zimmer's sales continued to increase.

Not that DePuy suffered any revenue loss. Despite the predictions of "experts," the demand for orthopedic products was more than enough to sustain not only two manufacturing companies in Warsaw, but new competitors as well. In fact, one was about to start up in the South.

AAOS Is Born and Modern Orthopedics Takes Form in Memphis

Fifty years before John Charnley created the first reliably successful hip replacement system, in the early 1900s, Memphis had fully recovered from the ravages of yellow fever epidemics that had nearly destroyed the city in the 1870s, and the area's economy was on an upswing.

For decades the city had been the world's largest inland cotton exporting center, and its prosperity had been enhanced before the close of the nineteenth century by *an increasing* demand for another local resource—the vast stands of timber that grew in the river valley. As the new century dawned, Memphis was undeniably the hardwood lumber capital of the nation, and business was booming for both hardwoods and cotton.

The city had also become an important railroad hub—the only railroad bridge over the Mississippi River between St. Louis and New Orleans was at Memphis—and it remained a busy river port. Eighty years later, it would become the home for Federal Express whose largest initial client was one of founding manufacturers of orthopedic products—Richards Manufacturing.

But, as the new century was finding its legs, Memphis was the kind of place a talented young southern doctor might find inviting.

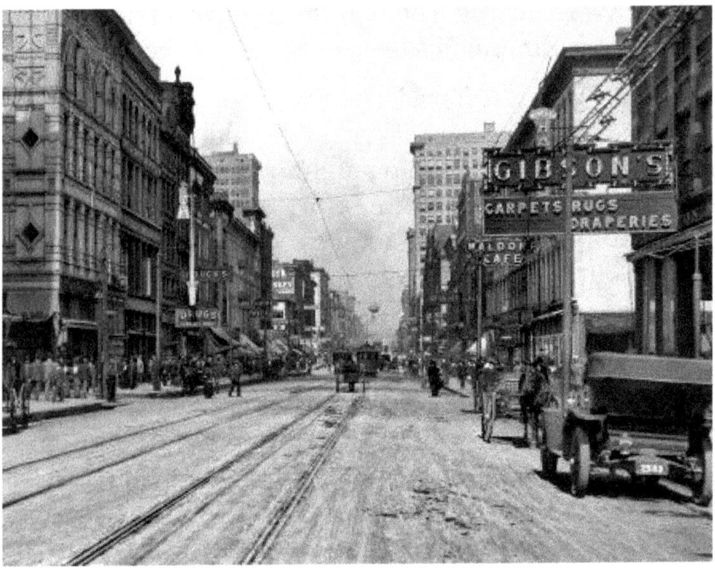

City of Memphis Downtown circa 1910
Source: Memphis City Government

Dr. Willis Cohoon Campbell – The First President of American Academy of Orthopaedic Surgeons (AAOS)

Dr. Willis Cohoon Campbell arrived in the city in 1906 just two years after receiving his medical degree from the University of Virginia, and it is probable that he had already decided that this was where he would open his own practice. Memphis was the largest city within a 200-mile radius, it was prosperous, and the young doctor would not be far from his hometown of Jackson, Mississippi.

However, Campbell did take a while to settle on a career. He first tried general practice and, briefly, pediatrics, but after a few years he began to think seriously about orthopedics. At that time, there were few orthopedic surgeons in the South, and Memphis was no exception. A new technology may also have influenced his decision—the discovery and use of X-rays.

Wilhelm Roentgen had discovered the potential of X-rays in 1895 when he made an X-ray photograph of the bones in his wife's hand, and by May of the following year Italian doctors were using the technology to find bullets in wounded soldiers. Bone structures were clearly visible in the X-ray films, and this meant that doctors no longer had to diagnose bone injuries and joint problems by touch alone.

Once Campbell chose to pursue a career in orthopedic surgery, he acted decisively. In 1909 he suspended his practice and traveled to Vienna to study under Adolph Lorenz, a leading orthopedic physician renowned for his methods of treating congenital hip dislocations, especially in children.

Lorenz had been a guest at the AMA's 1903 annual meeting and made regular visits to the United States, conducting lectures on his work. After working with

Lorenz, Campbell did further training with specialists in London, New York, and Boston before returning to Memphis in 1910 to begin a new medical practice, this time in orthopedics.

It turned out to be an auspicious time, as American medicine was about to undergo profound changes. Although Campbell had received his medical degree from a university, many doctors in his day entered practice with little formal education: some learned about medicine as apprentices to local physicians, while others enrolled in proprietary schools, institutions in which the school owners, usually local doctors, would lecture on various medical topics. Against this backdrop, it was not surprising that the quality of medical practice in the country varied greatly, and this inconsistency became a concern of the American Medical Association.

Many AMA members believed the fault lay with the training doctors received, and the logical first step was to find out how good, or how bad, medical education actually was. This would not be an easy task, however, and they decided to look for help outside the organization.

At the urging of the AMA's Council on Medical Education, the new Carnegie Foundation for the Advancement of Teaching agreed to fund a survey of American and Canadian medical schools, and Abraham Flexner was selected to lead the project.

Flexner was a progressive Kentucky educator and essayist who had recently published a controversial book highly critical of teaching methods at Harvard, where he had done postgraduate work. Although Flexner was not part of the medical fraternity, the director of the Foundation apparently liked what the educator had written. Flexner's findings would certainly be unvarnished. The results of the study were published in 1910 in *Medical Education in the United*

States and Canada, later known simply as "The Flexner Report."

As part of his research, Flexner visited and evaluated about 155 medical schools of all sorts, and many of these were found to be so wanting in the basics of medical education that they were forced to close. The report's description of a Knoxville school was typical: "The catalogue of this school is a tissue of misrepresentations from cover to cover." Other schools fared better, and in 1911 two proprietary schools in Memphis merged to form the University of Tennessee Medical School in Memphis.

That same year, Campbell applied for a position with the new school. He was not only accepted—he was asked to organize its Department of Orthopedic Surgery. Campbell quickly agreed and became the school's first professor of orthopedic surgery, holding that position until his death in 1941. He also continued to practice surgery and became "one of the pioneers in the development of arthroplasties," especially knee surgery.

Perhaps because of his early pediatric experience, Campbell was deeply concerned with the plight of children who had been crippled by orthopedic disease or injury, and in 1919 he helped found the Memphis' Crippled Children's Hospital, one of the first of its kind. This was followed four years later by the Hospital for Crippled Adults, established by Campbell and some of his friends and colleagues.

Always a strong supporter of advancing the profession of medicine, Campbell was one of the founders of the American Academy of Orthopaedic Surgeons and became its first president in 1933. He also found time to share his knowledge and experience with a wider audience, authoring numerous journal articles, a popular monograph (*Orthopedics of Childhood*), and *Orthopedic Surgery)*, a 1930 textbook.

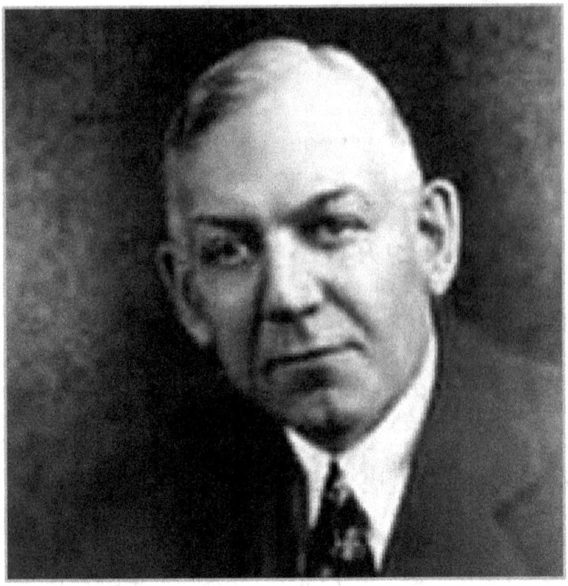

Dr. Willis Cohoon Campbell

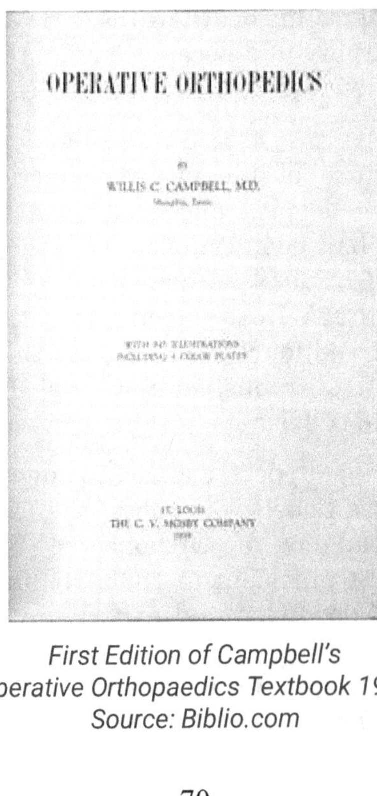

OPERATIVE ORTHOPEDICS

WILLIS C. CAMPBELL, M.D.

THE C. V. MOSBY COMPANY

First Edition of Campbell's
Operative Orthopaedics Textbook 1939
Source: Biblio.com

In 1939, near the end of his career, he also published *Operative Orthopedics*, which became the preeminent book in its field. Periodically updated and revised, the book would remain a classic: in 2007, the four-volume eleventh edition of *Operative Orthopedics* became available.

But it was for the clinic that bears his name that Campbell became most widely known. The Willis C. Campbell Clinic opened in December 1920 to offer specialized orthopedic care and to provide training in orthopedic surgery for doctors just out of medical school. It was so successful that four years later the clinic was able to establish postgraduate fellowships that guaranteed a level of expertise equal to what would soon be mandated by the American Board of Medical Specialties.

Determined to have only the best physicians in his new clinic, Campbell recruited the best medical school graduates. Three early enlistees were James Spencer Speed, Joseph Hamilton, and Joseph I. Mitchell, a Memphis native and graduate of the new medical school.

Speed had received his degree from the Johns Hopkins Medical School, but because he had no orthopedic training, he was initially reluctant to join the staff. Campbell convinced him that after a year of working under Campbell's personal supervision that he would be able to perform orthopedic surgeries on his own.

Hamilton's training was as an internist (an expertise that helped the clinic deal with various postoperative problems), and Mitchell's residency had been at the prestigious Mayo Clinic. Mitchell would later prepare many of Campbell Clinic's publications as well as author his own journal articles. By the beginning of the 1930s Campbell Clinic was widely recognized as one of the top orthopedic clinics in the country.

It was also an important asset to the region. There were few hospitals and little specialized medical care in the sparsely developed hinterlands, and this made Memphis the obvious choice for patients with any non-routine medical problems, including those that required orthopedic surgery. Moreover, a large percentage of local physicians were graduates of the University of Tennessee Medical School, where Campbell was still department head.

As a market for orthopedic goods, the South was not unlike the rest of the nation. Manual labor, which was the rule, guaranteed occasional broken bones, and quality splints meant quicker and better healing. Congenital skeletal problems could now also be treated by medical devices. Physicians understood this, and so also did DePuy Manufacturing in Warsaw. Wherever there were broken bones and malformations, and physicians to treat them, there was also a market for orthopedic products. And to reach the greatest number of markets throughout the nation, DePuy divided its sales force into different geographical regions, and Mississippi and Tennessee were assigned to one of its salesmen, J. Don Richards.

CHAPTER FOUR: RICHARDS MANUFACTURING

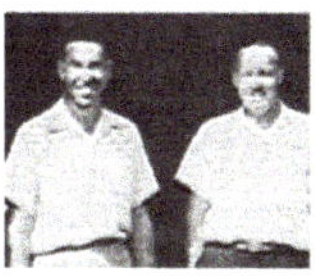

Harry Twiss and J. Don Richards, circa 1962

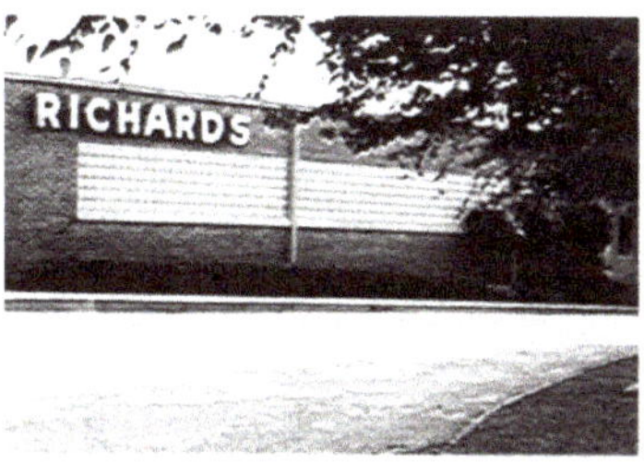

Richards Manufacturing on Brooks Road, Memphis, Tennessee, circa 198[illegible]

Sam Walton's original Walton's Five and Dime

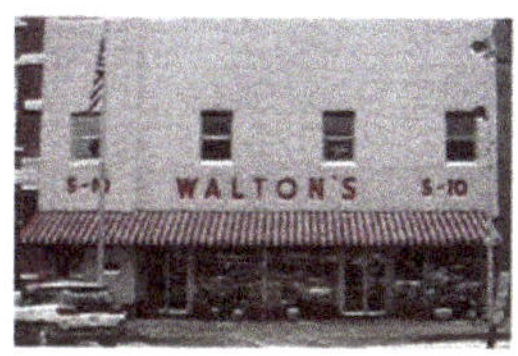

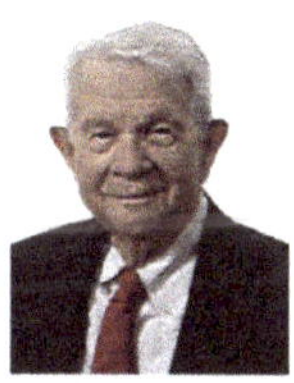

Society of Entrepreneurs and L.D. Beard

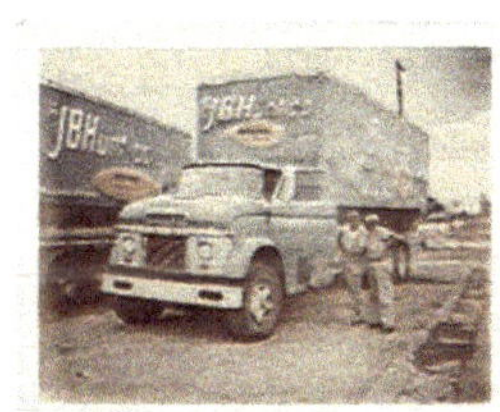

J.B. Hunt

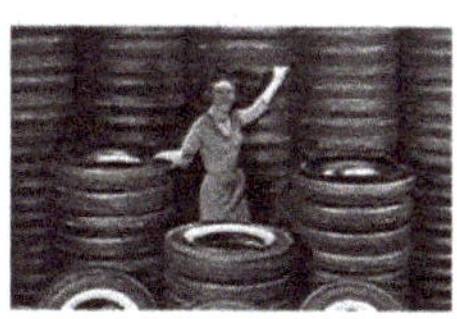

The Firestone Tire and Rubber Company

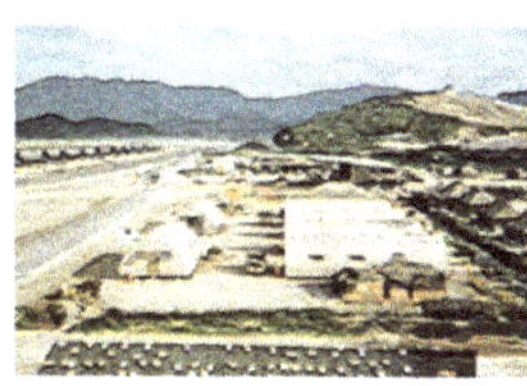

Air Force Base, Pusan South Korea

Don Richards was born on a farm near Warsaw, Indiana, and he had close family ties to DePuy's only business competitor, Zimmer Manufacturing. Richards' mother was the sister of J. O. Zimmer, and it was from him that Richards had first learned about the orthopedic business. With such connections, no doubt the young man could have done very well had he stayed in Warsaw, but it did not work out that way.

Richards' sales route took him through Brookhaven, Mississippi, a town due east of Natchez, in the heart of the Mississippi Delta. It was there that he met, fell in love with, and soon married, a young woman named Euna Brister.

Richards would later tell how he had explained to Euna, before they married, that because he was planning to go into business for himself they would have to move "up north." She was fine with that, she said, and was willing to move as far north...as Memphis. This was certainly not what Richards had in mind, but her notion of "north" apparently prevailed because in 1934 the couple moved to Memphis, where he opened the nation's third orthopedic manufacturing facility.

Richards Manufacturing Company started out in a rented building at 756 Madison Avenue, a few blocks east of downtown, next to a dry cleaners. It was not a large enterprise, but the choice of location made sense: Campbell Clinic and John Gaston Hospital were just down the street.

Predictably, the company's first products were splints, cast materials, and soft goods such as rib belts and arm slings, and its first buyers included the local hospitals, Campbell Clinic, and, after it opened, the orthopedic section of Kennedy Hospital.

An early specialty product was the Campbell-Boyd pneumatic tourniquet, a device which worked along the same lines as the inflatable cuffs used to take blood pressure measurements. The tourniquet was specifically designed for use by the Campbell Clinic and was sold only to the clinic.

Memphis' newest business got off to a good if modest start, relying on a handful of employees. Lelia Jones was hired as company seamstress (she personally sewed each belt and sling), and other initial employees were Jimmy Brower, who made the splints, and Pete Porch, who worked as a metal polisher.

C.C. "Smitty" Smith became the company's first salesman in 1938. Richards at this point was much smaller than either DePuy or Zimmer, but these three companies formed the foundation of the future orthopedic industry in the U.S.

Due to what can only be described as tragic reasons, the orthopedic business was about to boom. World War II brought an unprecedented demand for orthopedic products, and the U.S. government was soon buying large quantities of pins, plates, wires, slings and other devices from Richards, as well as from DePuy and Zimmer.

Richards may have had a unique advantage, at least in terms of feedback from doctors and even patients. In 1943, the Army opened a new general hospital in Memphis, and within three years it would become the largest such facility in the United States, with some 6,000 patients by war's end. Named in honor of a Spanish-American War surgeon, Kennedy Hospital would be taken over by the Veterans Administration in 1946.

Even after the war ended, Richards continued to enjoy dramatic growth as demand for new and better products continued to increase, and by 1950 Memphis would have its second orthopedic manufacturing company.

Among the new sales personnel that Richards hired during the war was Frank Wright, and in 1944 he became its Memphis area sales representative. A few years later, history—at least the piece of history that relates how orthopedic salesmen often have greater ambitions—was about to repeat itself.

Frank had learned from doctors that patients in leg casts frequently reported chronic back pain, which was attributed to the hard steel heel located at the foot of the cast, and Wright thought he saw a solution: replace the steel heel with a walking heel made of rubber.

He left Richards in 1950, patented his rubber heel device, and formed Wright Manufacturing Company to produce the heel. In later years, its product line would expand, making it a direct competitor with Richards and other manufacturers.

Another U.S. manufacturer, one which was not yet in the orthopedic business, but which would one day become the largest of them all, also experienced a surge in sales during the war. Its chief product was the Stryker Turning Frame, invented in the late 1930s by Dr. Homer Stryker while he was taking a course in surgery at the University of Michigan.

The frame made it possible to safely move bed-ridden patients suffering from spinal injuries. Near the end of the war Stryker also invented an oscillating saw which could cut through body casts without damaging the skin below. He applied for a patent on this in 1945, and it was granted a year later.

Notwithstanding the ever-increasing interest in his products, Stryker considered his inventions as merely a part of his regular practice, and it was not until 1946 that he incorporated his "sideline" as the Orthopedic Frame Company. That same year he hired as general manager a man who would also leave his mark on the industry, albeit at another manufacturer.

Harry Treace

Harry Tilson Treace was born in Leesville, Ohio, just south of Canton and about 80 miles due west of Pittsburgh and, as a young man, became the principal engineer and designing partner for a Kalamazoo, Michigan orthopedist named Homer Stryker, M.D.

In 1948, Homer Stryker, M.D. founded the Orthopedic Frame Company, the predecessor firm to Stryker Corporation. Harry was a gifted designer as well as a manager for Stryker. He and Dr. Stryker would invent and patent numerous medical devices together. In fact, Treace soon made modifications to Stryker's original cast saw design and in 1948 applied for a patent on his changes. The patent was granted, and he assigned it to Orthopedic Frame Company.

Treace also was allowed to buy stock in the firm. How many shares Treace purchased is not known, but the author of *The Stryker Story* believes it was "sizable." As part of the deal, Stryker apparently reserved the right to have first refusal if Treace decided to sell his shares.

Although both men contributed to the growth of the company, they did not always agree on how the company should be run. For example—this according to Treace's own handwritten notes—he was dismayed by Stryker's handling of a dispute with J.O. Zimmer, whose company had come out with a cast saw similar to Orthopedic Frame Company's device. Treace's account of this episode differs from that reported years later by Marshal Morrison, a long-time Stryker employee. Treace wrote:

"This story also is incorrect. Zimmer came out with and offered for sale a poorly designed Lucks Bone Saw with oscillating attachment. Homer and I went to Warsaw for a pow wow with J.O. Zimmer. The idea was to bring legal action if they didn't stop. J.O. sweet-talked Stryker into taking a small royalty [paid to him, not the company]. I wasn't pleased with the sell-out."

Partly because of such differences, the business relationship between Stryker and Treace was not to last, and again there are differing versions of exactly how the split came about. By 1954 it was obvious *to Treace* that Stryker was planning for his son Lee to take over the running of the company, and Treace began to look for other business opportunities that would let him use his talents.

The timing turned out to be fortuitous because Don Richards happened to be actively looking for an investor in his company. The two men met, and it did not take long for them to reach an agreement. Treace sold his Orthopedic Frame Company shares back to Stryker, bought a 40% interest in Richards Manufacturing Company, became its vice president and sales manager, and moved to Memphis.

Treace's impact at Richards was immediate and profound. In just his first two years with the company, he was responsible for the introduction of not one but two revolutionary medical devices—the Shea's stape ear implant made from Teflon and the compression hip screw, a device that significantly improved the treatment of hip fractures in the elderly.

Until then, the standard surgical procedure to repair a hip fracture was to nail the femur into the ball of the hip and secure it with screws fastened into a plate. Surgeons frequently used the Jewett nail, named for Dr. Eugene Jewett, who developed it in the 1940s. This procedure would work fine at first, but problems would arise as the healing hip naturally compressed.

Treace's device screwed into the ball of the hip and could move backward enough to let the bone compress naturally. Treace filed for the patent in 1956, and it was soon in heavy demand although the Jewett nail would remain popular as well.

Richards' overall sales growth was also strong, and by 1960 its annual sales reached approximately $800,000.

This was only about a fifth of the dollar volume recorded that year by Zimmer, which had become the industry leader, but both numbers would soon be dwarfed as a result of surgical advances by Charnley and others.

The entire industry was about to be radically transformed. Of course, no one at Richards knew this in August 1960—not Don Richards, not Harry Treace, and certainly not a newly-hired 27-year-old shipping room clerk: L.D. Beard.

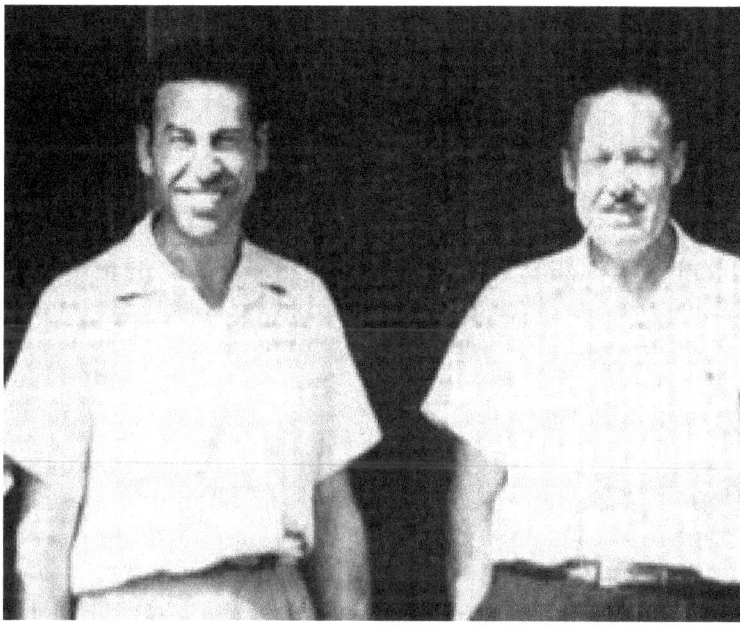

Harry Treace (left) and J Don Richards (right) circa: 1970

Leander Dallas Beard

As 1960 was winding down, the future president of Richards and who trained two generations of orthopedic and spine executives—whose managerial culture now infuses an entire industry—was wondering what he'd gotten himself into at Don Richard's young company on Brooks Road in Memphis.

To make matters worse, young Leander Dallas Beard (L.D. Beard) had turned his back on a stable, well-paying position at the largest private employer in the entire northern Mississippi and western Tennessee region—Firestone Tire and Rubber. Oh, and he'd also walked away from nine years of seniority or, as he would say in later years, "I was one year away from having a vested retirement there."

At Richards Manufacturing L.D. was standing in the lobby for, what he expected, would be his first day as Richard's new shipping manager. His college friend, Johnny Dean, was shipping manager before L.D. and was trying to move from shipping to sales. Johnny had personally recruited L.D.

So there L.D. was, on a Saturday morning in August 1960, with Johnny Dean when who should be passing through the lobby but Don L. Richards, himself, founder and President. Dean introduced him to L.D. and told Mr. Richards that L.D. was taking over his job in shipping.

Richards looked surprised, which in turn surprised L. D.

And what, asked Richards, was Dean, his current shipping department head, going to do?

"I'm going on the road to become a distributor in Ohio and Michigan," said Dean. Which also surprised Richards, who then asked when this transfer was taking place. Only when the new man was fully trained,

Dean assured him, which would take about two months.

"Oh, well," said Richards, "I just own the place. You don't have to tell me anything." And walked off.

Not like Firestone, thought L.D., where employment procedures were clear and formal.

Overtime, L.D. would come to learn that sarcasm was a Don Richards trait, but at the time all he could think was "What am I getting into?"

Later that day, back in the shipping department, Beard met Harry Treace, who was #2 at the company and had formerly been Homer Stryker's partner and co-founder of the Stryker Corporation in Michigan.

Treace was at least cordial.

During their first conversation Treace asked about L.D.'s service in the Air Force, Beard told him he had been trained as a radio operator, and Treace remarked that he had been a radio operator in a B-29 in World War II. L.D. volunteered that despite his training that radio was not something he really cared about.

"Neither do I," said Treace. "I don't care if I never see another one." It was not the last thing they were to have in common, but neither could know that at the time.

In the days that followed, L.D. became more dismayed when he saw how shipping and related operations were handled. Again, it was nothing like Firestone. In fact, it worse, even, than the Air Force.

The shipping system was, L.D. would recall, "one of the most inefficient operations I had seen." And part of it, he concluded, stemmed from his buddy Dean who'd been "a one-man show", processing and filling orders himself. No system.

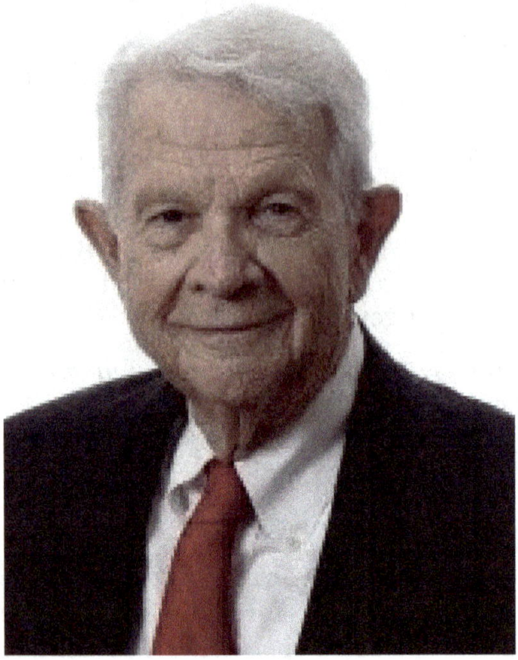

LD Beard / Courtesy of Society of Entrepreneurs and LD Beard

By November 1960, Richard Manufacturing's shipping department was in L.D.'s hands. And what he had was a real fixer upper. L.D. had a lot of work to do.

Yet, Richards Manufacturing was fairly typical of medical device companies in the late 1950s and early 60s.

In retrospect, it was obvious what L.D. would do. He would bring the logistics skills and best practices he learned at Firestone, the U.S. Air Force and, most critically, his own ability to analyze and break-down operational problems in a way that created new systems and taught the employees who ran them, how to operate an orthopedic/spine medical device business with both logistical precision and world class medical standards.

Within a decade, L.D. had Richards running like a modern medical device company, but more importantly, he was training a corps of young executives—notably E. Ron Pickard, who would eventually be the greatest of all medical device executives—a man whose legacy to the industry, to physicians and patients is almost beyond description.

L.D. Beard was part of a generation of hardscrabble entrepreneurs that emerged after World War II in the American South. This generation, forged by the economics of the American South post-Civil War, would transform retailing, trucking, food processing and, yes, orthopedic and spine medicine.

For most of the 100 years after the Civil War, which had destroyed the American south economically, the southern U.S. was significantly poorer than the rest of the country. The south's economic gap was neither strictly agricultural (although the south from 1860-1940 was predominately agrarian) nor racial. Wages of black and white farm laborers were virtually identical and farm labor wages were closely linked to wages in sawmills and textiles—the two largest Southern industries.

The south relied extensively on timber, cotton, and other agricultural products for its economic health prior to the 1960s, when a group of entrepreneurs emerged in Arkansas and Tennessee.

Sam Walton, born in 1918, while not the first, is the most famous of these hardscrabble entrepreneurs, each of whom founded their companies—incredibly—within a few miles of each other.

For Sam Walton, rural poverty was not a bug, it was a feature. Location, location, location are the three secrets to success in the retail business, so the saying goes. Sam Walton opened his first store in a remote, economically depressed and sparsely populated Ozark town—Rogers, Arkansas, population 4,900. Walton had another retailing secret in mind—namely supply the lowest priced consumer goods possible. To do that,

Walton famously innovated retailing operations, cutting inventory, labor and transportation costs and passing those savings to the consumer. Today we call that logistics management. But in 1962, in Rogers, Arkansas, it was entrepreneurism matching the hardscrabble life of his customers.

Walmart is the largest retailer in the world today.

Six miles south of Walmart, in Lowell, Arkansas, J.B. Hunt, the son of sharecroppers started a trucking company in 1961, one year before Sam Walton opened his first store up the road.

Hunt's innovation was to pay his drivers as low as possible which—ironically, put more money in each driver's pocket. Lower prices let Hunt schedule more freight. Of course, Hunt landed the Walmart contract.

Hunt's greatest innovation, one that transformed the global logistics business, was multi-modal (ships, trains, and trucks) container shipping. In 1980 inventory and transportation costs were 18% of the U.S. economy. Because of multi-modal shipping, inventory and transportation costs dropped to 8.5% of the U.S. economy. JB Hunt trucking grew to become the third largest shipping company in the world.

Five miles south of JB Hunt, John Tyson in Springdale, Arkansas, founded a company that, today, supplies one-fifth of the beef, chicken, and pork in the United States. John and his sons were also hardscrabble entrepreneurs who figured out how to squeeze costs out of the meat processing system by vertically integrating the entire system of growing and processing meat. Tyson also introduced the first ice-pack processing line.

And 200 miles southeast of Tyson Foods in Little Rock, Arkansas, Frederick Smith founded Federal Express in 1971. Also in Little Rock was the company that helped to fund these companies—Stephens Group—also founded by, you guessed it, hardscrabble bankers who started their business in the depths of the Great

Depression by selling near-bankrupt state bonds and bibles in the South.

That's a story for another day.

Frederick Smith, the founder of FedEx, the quintessential logistics company who created the concept of the overnight package delivery, started operations in 1973, 170 more miles east of Little Rock in Memphis Tennessee.

And it is in Memphis that we come to the Richards Manufacturing and L.D. Beard—a man who shares the same formative upbringing and training as the more famous people mentioned above—but whose impact on the business of supplying orthopedics and spine medical products around the world was no less transformative.

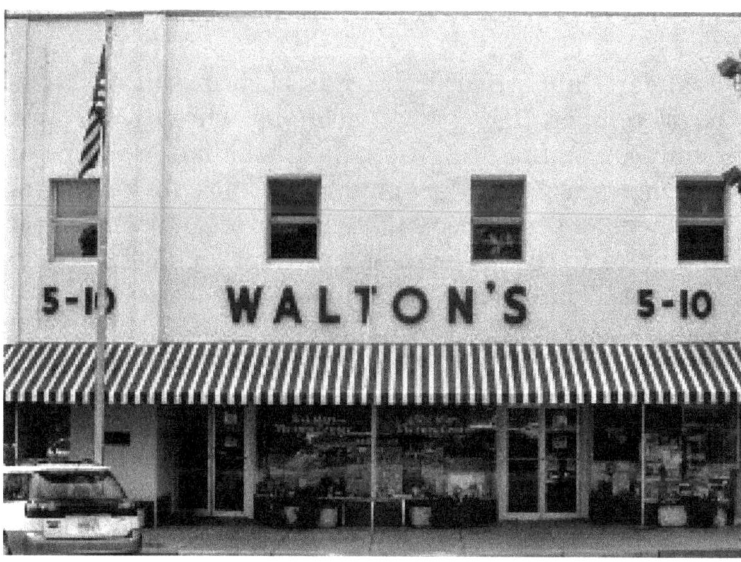

Sam Walton's original Walton's Five and Dime
Source: Wikimedia Commons and Bobak Ha'Eri

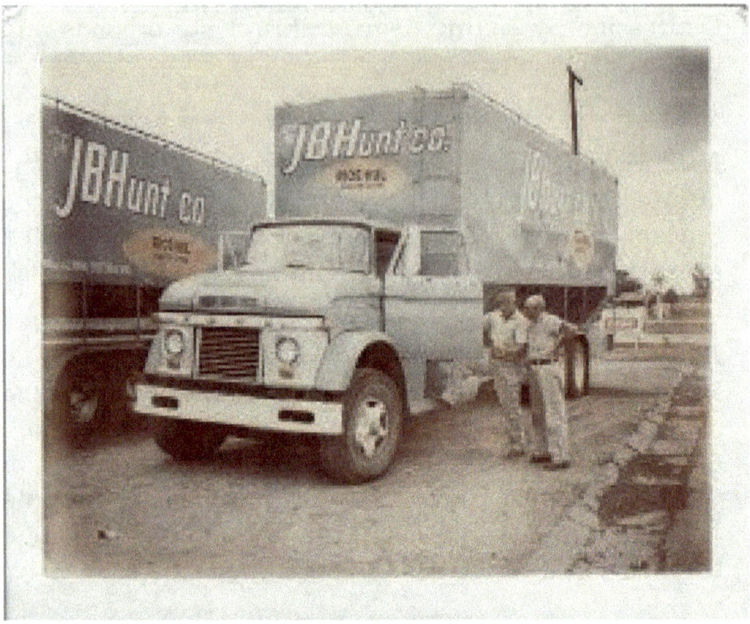

Courtesy of J.B. Hunt

Leander Dallas Beard, Jr., was born in Dallas, Texas on December 13, 1932, to a family whose roots were firmly in Tennessee. "Usually Christmas and during summer vacation, we would come back to see all the relatives in Tennessee." Remembers L.D. "We'd go from one place to the other seeing my mother's and father's relatives. That was every summer and Christmas."

L.D's father, known as "Dal" always owned a decent car; none of L.D.'s Tennessee relatives had one. They were that poor. Both his father and uncle sent money to their older sister in Tennessee so that her daughter would have clothes to wear for high school graduation. L.D.'s mother's relatives also struggled as tenant farmers. To L.D.'s Tennessee relatives, the Texas Beards must have seemed like rich folk.

In 1943, the Texas Beards decided to head back to West Tennessee. Dal found a job at the Milan Arsenal and L.D. started a new school at Moore's Chapel, a small community in Gibson County on the road between Milan and Trenton.

L.D. discovered very quickly that small town Tennessee schools are nothing like a Dallas, Texas schools. “To fit in, to be one of the guys, you had better not study or earn good grades or put on airs. If I used a word like ‘logical’, L.D. recalled, "I was accused of using a big word.” The lesson was clear, exert the least amount of effort in school necessary to earn the minimum passing grades. “I didn’t have to excel, but I knew I had to pass because if I didn’t pass my dad would have put me on a construction crew some place.” L.D. was 11 years old.

When he wasn’t in school L.D. worked. Farmers in Gibson County raised a lot of fruits and vegetables, and there were seasonal jobs aplenty. “During the summer, they had big pack sheds where the farmers would bring in their produce, starting with cabbage early in the year. I would work in the pack shed, 11 years old, and make 35 cents an hour, which I thought was great.”

When he was about 13 or 14 years old, L.D.’s father moved the family to Memphis to be part of the post-war building boom. During L.D.’s school years, the family moved often and L.D. would eventually attend 7 different schools in 11 years.

His final school was Whitehaven High School in Memphis, which, he remembers, was wonderful educational environment: “t had, really, at that time, a cadre of teachers who had been there for a long time. They were really great teachers. No matter what class you were, I mean what your economic status or whatever was, you were accepted very well there.”

Despite his natural curiosity and intelligence, L.D. was an indifferent student. In fact, to hear him tell it, he never studied: “My dad would say, ‘I thought I remember buying you some books at the beginning of the school year, and I haven’t seen them since then. Where are they?’”

By his senior year, L.D. was working part-time at the Hogue and Knott grocery store on the corner of Park Avenue and Highland Street. Saturday nights he sometimes had to work until the early morning hours of Sunday, but that was okay by him. Finding a job was always easy for L.D. New employers quickly spotted his talents and energy.

L.D. graduated from Memphis's Whitehaven high school in 1950.

Firestone Tire and Rubber

That same year L.D. registered with the local employment office, which soon scheduled an interview for him with Firestone. "I took the tests and filled out the application, and the comptroller was interviewing me and asked me, 'Why do you want to work for Firestone?'"

He was hesitant, not knowing the right thing to say, but the interviewer prompted him: "Is it because you want a job, and we have one?"

"I said, 'Yes, sir. You're right.'"

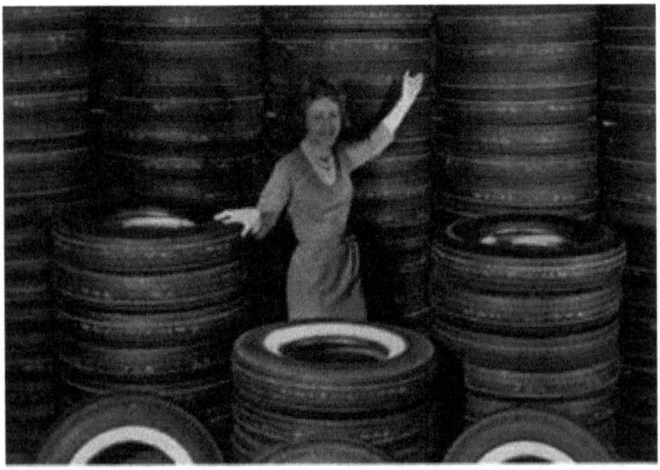

Courtesy of The Firestone Tire and Rubber Company

"You're hired," said the man.

The Firestone Tire and Rubber Company built its Memphis plant in 1936 on land previously occupied by a wood products company in the northwest corner of the city. Over time, the site would go through numerous expansions, eventually covering 35 acres near Thomas Street, and by the 1950s the company could advertise the factory as the "largest single tire producing unit in the world" with a workforce of approximately 4,000. Demand for its products was high and climbing, the pay and benefits were good, and in 1951 it was the kind of place where a young man just starting out might begin a career.

The 20 year old Beard, glad to have a full-time job, went to work for Firestone as a mail clerk in March 1951. His daily routine seldom varied: he and one other clerk would drive to the Thomas Street Post Office, bring back the company mail, sort it, and distribute it to various office around the massive plant. On their rounds, they would also pick up the outgoing mail, any bills of lading that needed signatures (for railway shipments), and any deposits. The latter two tasks required errands to offices in downtown Memphis before returning to Firestone to pick up any additional outgoing mail. A final trip to the main post office in downtown Memphis would mark the end of L.D.'s day. Not especially challenging tasks, but it meant a paycheck.

Shortly after he started at Firestone, his supervisor offered L.D. a promotion to the paymaster's office, which puzzled him. Delivering mail did not draw the attention of supervisors—until he found out why they wanted to keep him.

The comptroller's secretary explained. "She said, 'You know why they hired you, don't you?' And I said I thought they needed to carry all this mail around. "And she said, 'You know that test you took?' And I said yes.

And she said, 'You made the highest score on that that anybody has ever made.'"

The boy who had been satisfied with just sliding by in high school was surprised by her remarks although he did recall taking similar tests during his senior year at Whitehaven High School. In fact, the guidance counselor there had been astonished by his aptitude for numbers and had repeatedly urged him to pursue a career along those lines. At the time, he had dismissed the idea, but now, he thought, maybe there was something to that after all.

L.D. Beard was one of the youngest employees that had ever worked in the paymaster's office. Firestone's weekly payroll was close to $300,000, and each employee was paid in cash.

Earnings had to be verified and individual salaries counted and recounted, a sometimes tedious job but one at which L.D. excelled. The money was then put into envelopes, which workers in the paymaster's office would distribute to the employees, person by person, shift by shift. L.D. would finish the last shift around three o'clock Sunday morning and not have to report back to work until Tuesday.

It was also at Firestone that L.D. realized that he had a knack not only for dealing with numbers but for dealing with people as well. Over the next 18 months he would come to know and get along with just about everybody in the plant. There was only one exception: "I had one union steward who was determined to make my life miserable. If I didn't get out there right on the minute he thought I should, he'd file a grievance." But instead of overreacting to the hostility, as would many teenage boys, L.D. simply viewed it as part of the job: "We lived with it."

He liked the other employees he met, including the men on the work floor, and they liked him. "They all kidded me. I went off one weekend and got my hair cut off, and they rubbed my head and called me 'Fuzzy.' They all worked in the plant, and I'd come in with a dirty head. But it was a good job to have." L.D. would remain in the paymaster's office for nearly two years—$240 a month was a good wage—and would leave only because he had to.

The U.S. Air Force

The Korean War was still going on, and by December 1952, the local selective service board had classified L.D. as 1-A. "I had passed the physical and everything else, but I'd decided that I would rather be in the Air Force for four years than be in the Army for two." With the help of a couple Army recruiter friends, L.D. learned that he was on the U.S. Army induction list for the 29th of January, so on the 15th he enlisted in the Air Force for four years.

"About the second day in the Air Force I said, this is not going to be my career. My strategy was going to be to go four years unnoticed. I went through basic training. They gave you a whole series of aptitude tests—the highest score you could make was nine, and I made nines or eights on all of them, except radio operator. I made a five on that one."

Naturally, the Air Force next sent him to radio school at Keesler Air Force Base.

Radio operator was not how L.D. wanted to spend four years. His new strategy was to simply fail to meet the work standards. After he achieved a Morse Code score of 13 words a minute, he pretended he had reached his limit. His scheme might even have worked, but someone was checking his work.

A master sergeant confronted him, and L.D. would later recall the NCO's quiet demeanor: he was not angry, but he was emphatic: "We know what you're trying to do, and it's not going to work. We can't wash you out for cause, but we can put you on the front row of the classroom, and you'll be in there six weeks, and you'll have six NCOs watching you at all times."

L.D. stopped faking. In fact, he increased his code rate from 13 words a minute to 20 in one afternoon. "They didn't know whether to congratulate me or kill me."

Over his Air Force career, L.D.'s responsibilities steadily increased as his base assignments moved from Otis Air Force Base on Cape Cod to Tokyo, Japan, then a small air base near Pusan, South Korea and finally, in 1955, Barksdale Air Force Base outside Shreveport, Louisiana, where he would remain until he was discharged in 1957.

It was during his last posting that L.D. found his way into some training that might indeed help in his later career, although he was initially not interested in it at the time: "The squadron CO wanted to send me to leadership school because I was Airman First Class. I told him, 'Major Butts, the Air Force is wasting their money.'"

"It was probably in May of '56, or something like that, and the major was insistent."

He was up for promotion to Lieutenant Colonel, and he intended to send L.D. and another airman: "One of you will be number one, one of you will be number two, when you come out of leadership school, and that's going to look very good for me."

The leadership course lasted a couple months, and, as the major had predicted, L.D. and the other airman received the two highest grades.

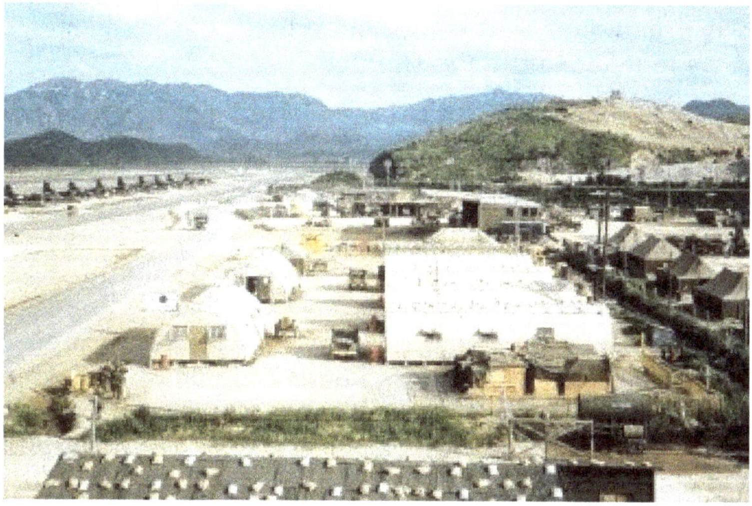

Air Force Base, Pusan South Korea
Source: Wikimedia Commons and U.S. Air Force

L.D. Finds His Way to Richards Manufacturing

When he left military service in early 1957 L.D. returned to Firestone and after a short stint back in the mailroom, L.D. was transferred to the cost accounting department. He finally had a job that was both challenging and rewarding. It exposed him not only to cost accounting but also to engineering whenever a new tire design was developed, L.D. would be involved in running the projected costs, an area in which he became proficient.

"I really got exposed to that part of the business and, of course, you start out with an engineering specification, and you just broke it down into all the various components, whether it was labor or material or whatever."

But this required more than simply working with numbers at a desk. "That work exposed me to a lot of systems because I had to get out in the plant, and I had to see what they were doing and how they were doing it. I had done that some before because they liked for me to take plant tours through."

"I don't know why, but they selected me to take plant tours through for people, visitors who were coming in, so I had already learned some of it, but I had to get out and learn the rest of it."

At the same time, L.D. was beginning to form some definite opinions about the operations he witnessed, especially the importance of having the proper equipment. Cost analyses for each product were done twice a year, using a comptometer, a kind of mechanical calculator originally developed in the 19th century, and a simple ink pen. In L.D.'s view, hardly the best equipment for the task. But there was at least one upside: using the comptometer took a lot of hours, which translated into considerable overtime pay.

When he went to work at Richards Manufacturing in Memphis, Tennessee, L.D. knew nothing about the company, its industry, its customers, or its products other than what his friend Johnny Dean had told him, which was not much. And the "orientation" he received from Dean was almost laughable. Indeed, decades later, L.D. would laugh whenever he described his introduction to his new job.

"I followed Johnny Dean around for the first couple of days there, and he was taking orders and doing different things he did, and at the end of two days, he said, 'Do you have any questions?' And I said, 'Yeah. What's an implant? And what's an instrument?' That was about the extent of my knowledge, really. I had no idea what they did or who they were except what Johnny had told me."

There is more than a little truth in the anecdote, but he soon learned.

When L.D. went to work for Richards in 1960, its product line consisted mainly of medical soft goods—sewn or molded items, including cervical collars, rib belts, slings, and splints—and specialty products designed by Treace, including Shea's stapes and his patented compression hip screw, both of which sold well.

And the operation was, in some ways, co-managed by Don Richards and Harry Treace, who split Richards' ownership 60/40, respectively—Treace being the junior owner. Don Richards was the president and Treace designed and developed products.

Before L.D. arrived, Johnny Dean had run all aspects of the shipping department and it was chaotic. "I knew I had to get some order into the system, which was very difficult to do. To keep from having to do all of the things that Johnny was having to do, and to also share some of the responsibility with some of the others in the department rather than try to be a one-man show, which I started doing. I hired one other person not too long after I came in."

Compounding L.D.'s task was Don Richards' style of management. Richards reviewed every piece of mail that came in and choose which orders to fill first, which created some difficulties for the shipping department.

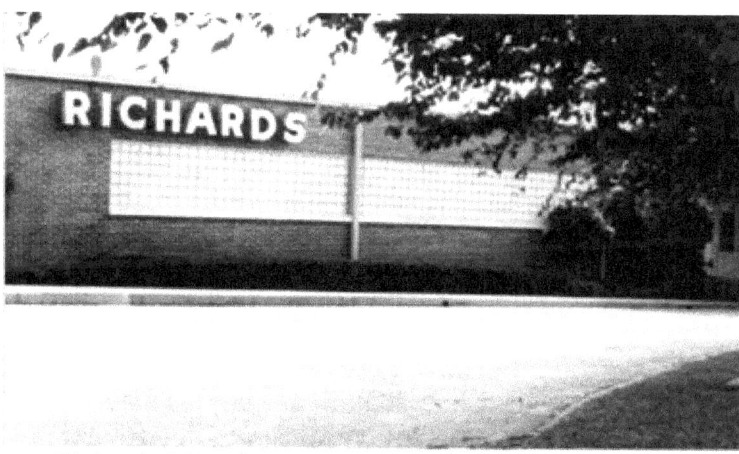

Richards Manufacturing on Brooks Road, Memphis, Tennessee, circa 1986

"We'd put shop orders on inventory that we needed because we also kept the inventory control back there. Well, if he'd looked at the mail three or four days in a row and the orders were light, he'd go back and cut the shop orders, so I'd have maybe 70 or something on order and 30 of them would come up, and I'd say, 'Where are all the rest?'"

"'Well, the boss came back and cut it.'"

"Every afternoon as we got these rush orders in for our hip nail, invariably, we'd go to the stock drawers, pull out what we had, start cutting them to different lengths as the customer had ordered, and get them out the door that afternoon. And it was absolutely chaotic. The inventory system and the whole system was absolutely chaotic. But it suited him, and the employees loved him."

Don Richards was certainly easy to spot: a robust man about six feet tall, he always wore a large Stetson hat, and a sport shirt buttoned all the way to the top. And because it was *his* company, he was not hesitant to express his opinions, chief among them was the urgency of keeping costs low.

Treace, on the other hand, focused on product development and, especially, quality. "He knew that quality would have to continue to improve in this business. There were no Food and Drug Administration controls or anything else. You just made it and put it out," L.D. would recall.

Sometimes, Don Richards' do-it-quick-and-cheap approach created problems. Not long after L.D. joined Richards, the company was awarded a bid from the military to manufacture a device called a Steinman Pin, a kind of guide pin used in surgery. There was a deadline on shipping, and the shipping department feverishly worked to package and ship the pins.

Don Richards decided to speed things along.

"We were packaging the pins in a clear, flexible plastic tubing and sealing it with an old heat sealer which trapped air in. The pins had to be packaged according to military specs, so many dozen in a package, and so many packages in another package, then waterproof paper and everything around them. So, Mr. Richards came back to try to speed things along. The young man I had hired was packaging, and he told Mr. Richards that he couldn't keep the air out of the pin packages."

Richards' solution was expedient: punch holes in every package.

"So, the young man did what his president told him to do. He punched a hole in every one of the Steinman Pin packages. When the Military inspector came out to the plant, the first thing he did was to drop one of the pin packages into a bucket of water and see if it leaked, which it did. He said this isn't going to pass, and I said, 'Well, none of them will then.'"

This was on a Thursday, and the inspector gave L.D. and his shipping staff until Monday to unpack and repack the items properly. They met the deadline, working night and day.

But that kind of seat-of-the-pants misdirection was much too frequent and made L.D.'s goal of creating a smooth running shipping and inventory department so difficult.

Problem by problem, L.D. was wrestling order out of chaos in Richard's shipping and inventory departments. Treace noticed and, in addition to his other tasks, asked L.D. to supervise Richard's middle ear implant production. These implants were all hand-crafted by two employees. L.D. was never sure why he was chosen to supervise the department, but he later guessed it was Treace's doing. The vice president began to act as a mentor to the young man, showing him all the various aspects of company operations.

As it was, it fit in with L.D.'s own management style, which had evolved from his experiences in the Air Force and at Firestone. "I could see how you broke things up into bite-sized pieces. And so I think I had learned that just from my experience observing at Firestone and observing in the Air Force that's how it's done—how they broke them into smaller pieces. I'd have regular meetings with the staff to bring out any kind of problems or anything they had."

Creating the First Orthopedic Device Packaging Line

Over lunch one day, Treace told L.D. that he thought the packaging, especially for a medical company, was "horrible," and L.D. quickly agreed. "Well," said Treace, "I think you have the flair and the ability to come up with a good packaging program. So, would you take that on?"

Treace wanted him to find a packaging show someplace and then go there and learn what he could. This was indeed new: L.D. had never done any travel on behalf of the company before. They also agreed not to tell Don Richards—trips cost money.

L.D. found a good equipment show, in Chicago, and he spent a day or two there looking at all kinds of packaging equipment. "It was just overwhelming to see what all could be done. And that's the first time I had even thought about it." It gave him some ideas he wanted to put into place.

By coincidence, on the airplane trip home, he sat next to Arthur Katz, who was part-owner of Paper Products Company in Memphis. Katz asked what he had been doing in Chicago, and L.D. told him.

Back in Memphis, Katz soon called on L.D., and the two of them exchanged ideas about how to improve the packaging system at Richards. L.D. liked Katz's ideas, and it was the beginning of a long-time business relationship. When L.D. left the company many years later, Katz was still calling on him.

Creating a Medical Inventory and Shipping Operations System From Scratch

As early as 1961, it was clear that the Madison Avenue location was simply inadequate, and the company purchased twenty acres on Brooks Road at the edge of the city as the site for a new plant and began developing plans for the new facility.

This was good news from L.D.'s perspective because at last there would be an opportunity "to design a shipping department that would work." He also was given the responsibility of coordinating the entire move.

By 1963, the plans for the plant were moving along—and just in time. Sales had more than doubled over the past two years, with a similar increase in the number of employees. The change was desperately needed.

The move was scheduled for a weekend—L.D. was determined they not miss a day of shipping if possible—and a few days before the actual move Treace found him at the new building.

"Well, where is your office?" asked Treace.

They happened to be standing near the executive offices and L.D. answered truthfully, that he had a desk in the shipping office. "That won't do," said Treace. "You take this office." The executive office next to him.

Treace noticed that L.D. was wearing the standard issue shipping room uniform and added: "And when you come in on Monday morning, wear a business suit."

Don Richards Dies Unexpectedly

Early in 1963, Don Richards had begun experiencing health problems. They did not appear all that serious, and he initially went to an osteopath for treatment, which didn't help. As the symptoms worsened, Richards went to a different doctor and his diagnosis was, correctly, Hodgkin's Disease. After the move to Brooks Road, Don Richards stopped working and was only able to visit the plant a few times.

Meanwhile, Treace was continuing to enlarge the sales force to keep up with rising demand for new orthopaedic products. Years later, looking at manufacturing and sales records, L.D. calculated the company's rapid growth rate: it worked out to more than a 25% compound annual growth rate—which strained even the new building on Brooks Road.

In March 1964 Don Richards died, and Harry Treace became CEO. As part of their agreement when Treace had bought into the company in 1954, each was given the right to buy the other's share in the event of death. It took about three months for Treace to raise the necessary cash and ten years after buying into Richards Manufacturing, Harry Treace was its sole owner.

One of Treace's first moves was to elevate L.D. Beard. L.D. would never forget how Treace broke the news.

"Let's go to lunch, L.D.," Treace said. And he took Beard to the Summit Club atop the Sterick Building. Another new experience: it was the first time L.D. had ever been in a private club.

Treace got right to the point. "I really appreciate the quiet way you go about your job. You get things done, and you don't make any noise about it or anything else. You just do it and get it done. I appreciate that. I have the company now. Everything has worked out, and what I'd like you to do is draw up an organizational chart and put yourself anywhere on it you want to be. Get back with me in about two or three weeks, and let's get it worked out."

This was far more than L.D. had expected. In fact, it was too much, and he was relieved a few days later when Treace offered him some guidance. Treace wanted to bring in William E. Fisher—who had been the company's auditor—as treasurer and second man in the organization. Bill, as he was called, would handle company finances, and Treace would continue to manage sales and marketing. L.D. was to become plant manager, handling all plant functions, including personnel, production, and purchasing.

L.D. Beard had only been at Richards four years!

Union

Richards Manufacturing was maturing and growing rapidly—riding the wave of hip replacement growth and the newly signed Medicare law, which brought millions of over 65 years old patients into the market for hip, knee, shoulder, hand and wrist, foot and ankle products.

In part because of Don Richards' illness and subsequent death, employees had had no pay raise in two years. They liked Don Richards a lot, but the new management team—Treace, Fisher, and Beard—were mostly unknown quantities.

This was especially true of Treace. "They viewed him as kind of standoffish, indifferent." The Richards employees decided to form a union.

When Treace and L.D. first heard about it, it was already a *fait accompli*. L.D. was working late one evening when one of the young men he had hired to work in the shipping department told him that he was going to quit, that he did not want to be part of a union. But Richards did not have a union, L.D. reminded him.

"You will have tomorrow," said the young man.

The next day, L.D. told Treace, who called a supervisors' meeting. None of had heard anything about a union. In fact, they laughed it off, thinking the young man had somehow gotten his facts confused.

"About an hour later the mail came in," recalls L.D., "and Harry laid a letter on my desk. It was from the International Association of Machinists saying they represented a majority of our bargaining unit employees and wanted to get together to discuss a contract."

The company's new management quickly retained a labor attorney and turned the matter over to him. They had a company to run. Besides, it might not be so bad.

At that time, Fisher and L.D. were in the process of selecting the company's first computer, and they were working with the computer people when they got the news: "Somebody stuck their head in the door and said everybody just walked out. The whole shop just walked out. I looked out across the street, and they had the picket signs and everything else out."

At that point it was a strike for recognition, and, as L.D. recalled, "it's hard to say that you have a 'good faith doubt' that they're representing the majority when they're all across the street.:

They contacted their labor attorney and began negotiating a contract. The company was willing to grant a significant pay increase—L.D. later recalled that it was in the neighborhood of 30% because they had not had one in so long—but the company was unwilling to concede on other issues. They felt they were being asked to surrender control of the company.

Negotiations turned bitter, and when the union struck again—according to L.D., breaking their promise not to strike while the mediator was out of town—the company began hiring replacements. The election was held, and the bargaining unit was recognized, but the company continued to hire replacement workers. Only when a union representative from New Orleans became involved did negotiations make any progress.

L.D. welcomed the breakthrough. "As soon as he sat down and started talking, I knew they'd run in someone who knew what he was doing. He just sat down and said, 'We're not going to have any problems. I've checked you people out. You have money. That's what it's going to be all about. We're not going to get into the emotional stuff, and so let's go ahead and negotiate a contract.'"

He was L.D.'s kind of man, polite but to the point—the point being to get the dispute settled. A contract was negotiated over the next two days, and both sides signed on. "I took it out to Harry Treace's home because he wouldn't even come in to the negotiations. He was totally emotional about it, too. He signed it, and we had a contract."

It turned out to be more than a standard win-win scenario. The company virtually doubled in size the following year, and L.D. was able to bring back many of the workers who had been replaced. Two would even become supervisors.

There was also a strange epilogue. It was only a one-year contract, and the following year negotiations again hit an impasse, partly over the issues of a dues check-off, which the company opposed. But by then some workers were not pleased with the idea of having a contract at all: before unionizing, many employees had become used to coming in and talking with L.D. about whatever they wanted to. Correctly, L.D. would say he was bound by the contract and could not negotiate with them individually, and this left them frustrated. In time, a number of employees even sent the company a list of people who had signed a petition to end the union. Rather than file decertification proceedings, L.D. simply filed away the list. No new contract was ever signed, and Richards became the largest manufacturer in the city without a union contract.

CHAPTER FIVE: ORTHOPEDIC MANUFACTURING BECOMES A GROWTH INDUSTRY

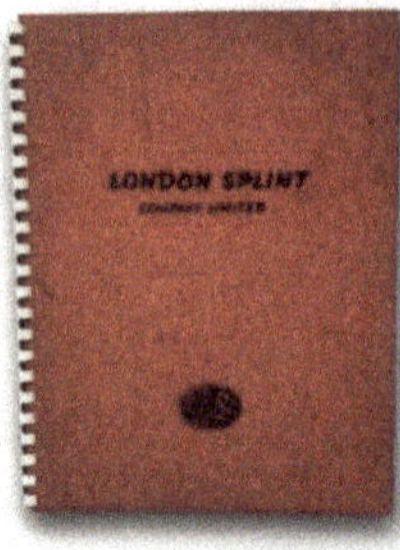

London Splint Company Catalog, circa 1958

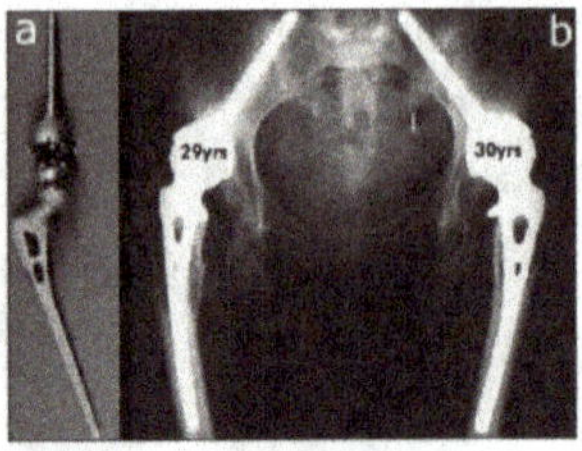

Franklin Sammann

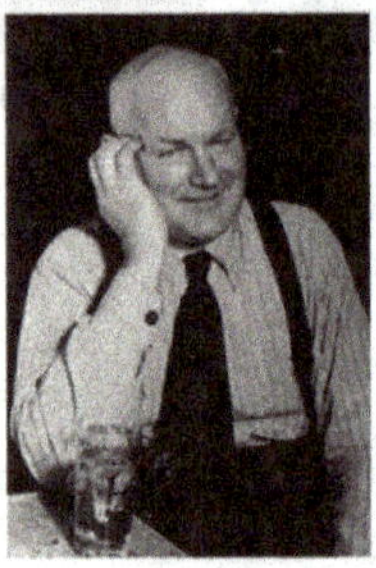

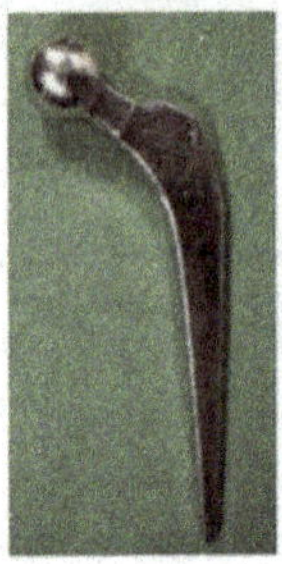

Ring metal on metal total hip

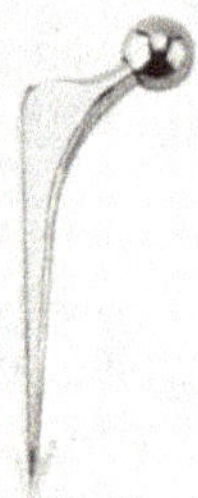

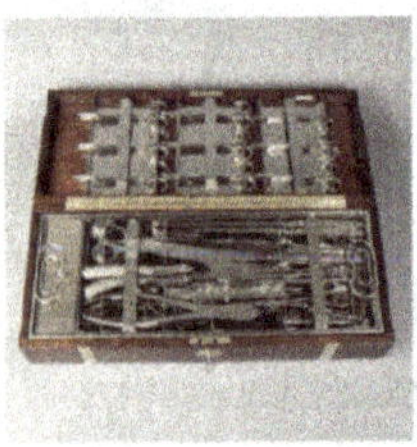

Down Brothers Instrument Tray circa 1960s

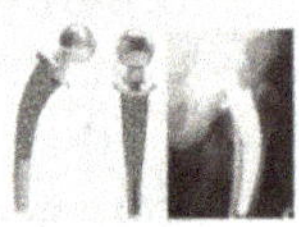

Biodynamics Hip by Howmedica

Exeter Hip

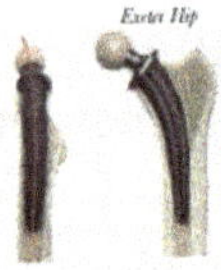

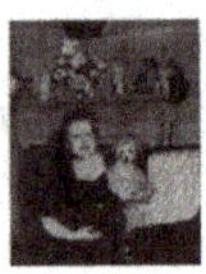

Mrs. Annette Hoopes, DePuy President circa 1964

By any measure, what Charnley accomplished in the late 1950s and early 1960s had transformed the treatment of hip disease, and the succeeding years saw an explosion of remarkable advances in orthopedic surgery and a sharp rise in the number of successful hip implants.

Surgery did not merely partner with science and engineering—the fields essentially merged, producing benefits that would have been unimaginable just a few years earlier.

It is no exaggeration to say that because of Charnley's breakthrough the once lame could now walk. But that was only the beginning.

Even though Charnley was clearly the leader in total hip replacement, he was not the only British surgeon conducting research in the area. Throughout the ensuing decade, McKee continued his work at Norwich, while three other groups developed their own distinct surgical techniques, each with a different combination of methods and materials.

While Charnley's name would be forever identified with his devices (and with their derivations, such as the Charnley-Müller prosthesis), these other systems would come to be associated with the specific locales in which they were developed instead of with the names of the surgeons who designed the techniques and new devices.

Hence, the Stanmore Group, the Redhill-Ring Group, and, not least, the group that gave its name to the Exeter Hip. And each of these in turn would go its own way in choosing materials and manufacturers.

Yet despite their differences, each group initially shared a common feature: research was led and controlled by surgeons, not by independent engineers or manufacturers. No doubt one reason for this was a factor that had no equivalent in the United States: Britain's National Health Service (NHS). Established in 1948, the NHS guaranteed every British citizen access to medical care, including surgery, and it supported research in a wide variety of fields while attempting to keep costs down. And research, from the NHS perspective, meant *medical* research conducted by surgeons. As at Wrightington, so also at other locales.

It was a system that produced some remarkable breakthroughs, but the role of the surgeon as director of all aspects of research and product development was not to last, and the first departure from this practice occurred at Exeter.

Whereas Charnley always maintained close control over every aspect of his research, including both the design and the manufacture of his implants, the Exeter team shifted much of the responsibility for design and testing to a university engineer and left control of the manufacturing process itself to the company actually producing the devices.

At that time, its supplier was The London Splint Company. Of course, there could be drawbacks with either method. If a surgeon-researcher became comfortable with specific techniques and materials that appeared to work satisfactorily, there was little incentive to develop alternative techniques or materials.

To be sure, there was usually quick response whenever difficulties arose—witness Charnley's actions following his unsuccessful efforts with PTFE—but the primary aim in such instances was to improve the system already being used. On the other hand, greater independence for manufacturers could create another set of problems, as Exeter's own experience would one day demonstrate.

Many of these differences in surgical techniques and implant design came about partly because total hip replacement surgery was still in its infancy in the 1960s. New devices that looked promising, whether coming from surgeons or engineers, might or might not work very well in practice, but as yet there was little in the way of uniform testing in either the U.S. or the U.K. Nor is this surprising.

Despite fundamental differences in how health care was delivered, the two countries were similar in one key respect: although research and testing of new *medicines* prior to their use by the public was routine, neither government mandated a testing regimen or approval of orthopedic devices prior to their use in actual surgery, and this remained true throughout the decade.

This absence of uniform testing protocols was not, however, due to any failure to appreciate the risks involved. Instead, it was mainly because of the inherent differences between administering medicine to a patient and surgically placing a prosthesis into the patient's body.

The pharmaceutical review model relies on randomized testing over a time period long enough to evaluate both beneficial and adverse effects, all the while controlling for independent factors that might influence the outcome. Double-blind studies are even better: these are trials in which neither the patient nor the doctor knows whether the medication being administered is actually the drug being tested, another drug, or a placebo. Moreover, if severely adverse effects are detected, or if a patient simply wishes to withdraw from the study, his or her participation in the trial can be halted.

Replicating this testing model within the context of hip replacement surgery was simply not possible.

"Dosage" such as it is in arthroplasty, could be carefully measured and monitored, but surgeons brought to their practices varying skill levels and product or technique familiarity. Further, it could take years to detect problems accurately attribute them to either surgical technique or implant material.

Double-blind studies were impossible because the surgeon would always know which technique and devices were being used.

Finally, there was also an ethical dilemma that troubled the medical profession right from the beginning of orthopedic implants. Although doctors must provide what they believe to be the best possible treatment for their patients, clinical trials may require that this standard be subordinated to a larger goal—namely, the future good of all patients.

In the early days of arthroplasty, it was not clear which approach was superior and individual surgeons had individual opinions as to superior treatment. How could a physician ethically withhold a treatment that he or she believes is in the patient's best interest?

Charnley had shown what was possible; the question now was whether another method would permit the surgery to be performed faster, easier, with less likelihood of infection, and with better long-term benefits to the patient.

Theories were plentiful, but for even the best researchers there was a jagged learning curve, and many advances were preceded by earlier failed attempts to improve upon Charnley's procedures and materials.

Many different joint replacement approaches emerged, affecting both patients and manufacturers. Conflicts raised their heads even before news of Charnley's success had crossed the English Channel.

The Stanmore Group

One team of researchers, centered at Stanmore on the outskirts of London, was the product of a collaboration between physicians John T. Scales and J. N. Wilson, both of whom practiced at Stanmore's Royal National Orthopaedic Hospital. The design team also included Ian Duff-Barclay, a biomechanical engineer for the British Petroleum Research Centre who had been assigned to work for the Institute of Orthopaedics at the University of London. Duff-Barclay was not working for Scales and Wilson, but *with* them, as evidenced by his co-authorship of numerous articles.

Their 1956 experiments resulted in "double-cup" acetabulum prosthesis. As the name implies, this device used two cups instead of just one. It was not the same double-cup device that Charnley initially used.

At Stanmore, an outer cup was first fixed into the hip socket by nails driven in by a pneumatic hammer specifically designed for this purpose. This was done to keep the nails from backing out and interfering with the movement of the prosthetic femoral head.

To further protect against such interference, a second, inner cup was also inserted and locked into position. This inner cup could be removed, if necessary, but the chief advantage of the system was that the acetabulum cup did not require cement.

Stanmore researchers also discovered that the acrylic resin in the cement, such as that used by Charnley at Wrightington, would degrade and begin to appear in patient urine just over a year after the implant.

A second difference from Charnley's procedure was that both components of the Stanmore prostheses—the femoral prosthesis and the acetabular cup—were made of metal, whereas Charnley's acetabular cup was a form of plastic. Stanmore's femoral stem was also round-tapered and slightly angled to make its insertion into the femur's marrow cavity easier.

In testing various metals thought to be suitable for prostheses, Stanmore researchers concluded that a cobalt-chromium alloy offered the best wear qualities. Titanium had showed the worst test results—devices made of titanium failed soon after testing started—and stainless steel did not perform much better. Consequently, Stanmore surgeons used chrome-cobalt for both the cup and the femoral stem, and the Stanmore Total Hip Replacement was patented in both the United Kingdom and the United States in 1966.

Stanmore's other major contribution during the early years of orthopaedic implant surgery was a change in how various innovations moved from theory to practice.

By working as a design team that included an engineer as well as a surgeon, the group developed a new way of conducting biomedical engineering in the field.

Expertise in chemistry and physics, especially in the development of implant materials, was not merely as important as surgical skill—the two fields had become intertwined.

The Redhill-Ring Group

A second group began its work at Redhill General Hospital in southwest England under the direction of Peter A. Ring, who had become interested in hip replacement surgery while holding a research fellowship at the Royal College of Surgeons from 1954 to 1957.

Three years later, he began his own research at Redhill, working along the same lines as Charnley, including the use of a cemented plastic cup with a metal femoral prosthesis. Like Charnley, he also noticed that the plastic would break down and that the resulting particles would irritate the surrounding tissue.

In revision surgery—subsequent corrective surgery that was sometimes required when a device did not seat properly or otherwise did not perform as intended—he also discovered that the cement did not bond the cup firmly enough to the hip socket. Further experiments convinced him that attaching the cup with a long threaded shaft, along with careful positioning of the femoral prosthesis, would produce a sufficient bond without the use of any cement.

Ring eventually became convinced that the best material for a metal prosthesis was cobalt-chrome alloy, which was also the material settled on at Stanmore. The shape of the femoral stem was similar to the one used by Moore in the U.S., but Ring's device had openings in it that allowed bone material to grow into and around the shaft after insertion. Neither component of the Redhill prosthesis used cement for fixation or bonding.

The overall design remained unchanged until 1967, when a series of changes were introduced, each responding to a deficiency in its predecessor.

That year the Redhill group redesigned the acetabular cup and the screw that held it in place in order to reduce fatigue fractures that resulted from weight and other stresses over time. When problems also arose with the femoral stem—it originally had been very narrow—the stem was redesigned to eliminate a tendency to tilt.

Unfortunately, this 1969 change had its own downside: it produced "prosthetic migration," the movement of the prosthesis from its original position. To resolve this new problem, Redhill researchers created three different sizes of femoral stems in 1971, each of which used a "straight-stem" design originally developed by Moore. These final changes seemed to eliminate this problem, although there would be additional modifications, and Ring's total hip replacement system would not finally become standardized until 1981.

Switching from metal-on-metal to metal-on-plastic was one thing, but Ring was unwilling to adopt Charnley's use of cement.

In fact, a number of disadvantages associated with cement persuaded him to avoid it entirely. Cement made any subsequent removal surgery more difficult, and the likelihood that hip replacements would loosen also tended to be greater with patients who had cemented implants than with those whose implants had been done without cement. The problem was not so much with the loosening itself as with the presence of particles that inevitably wore off the plastic cup as a consequence of the loosening. These particles, in turn, could increase toxicity problems.

Ring also was concerned about two problems connected with the acrylic cement itself. The first was a consequence of mixing the polymer: the chemical reaction produced heat and pouring the heated cement into the bone might cause tissue damage. Secondly, Ring believed that later infections in patients might be due to the amount of cement in the body. For both of these reasons, Ring decided to stay with uncemented fixation.

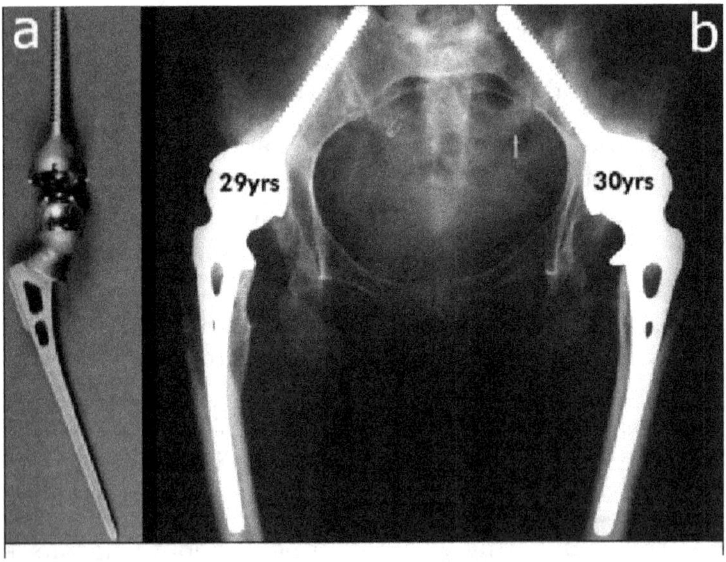

Ring metal on metal total hip / Source: Joseph Daniel

The Exeter Group

The third research group, this one in Exeter, a few miles south of London, first began working on hip replacements in 1965.

The Exeter team consisted of an engineer, Clive Lee, and a surgeon, Robin Ling. Lee held an engineering degree and had worked for Rolls Royce on jet engines in the early 1960s, and Ling had specialized in orthopedics at the Royal National Orthopaedic Hospital at Stanmore a few years before Scales and Wilson began their research there.

When Ling had arrived in Exeter in 1963, he had initially sought a position in pediatric orthopedics, but the area was already filled with specialists. He then turned to his second choice: trauma injuries. It was a decision with far-reaching consequences.

Throughout the mid-1960s, thanks to the work of Charnley and others, the demand for hip replacement surgery continued to increase, and the question for Ling and Lee—as it had been for Ring—was which kind of device to use in their surgeries. Initially, they used a metal-on-metal prosthesis, but by 1969 the group was encountering problems with prosthesis loosening, which they attributed to excessive friction found in the metal-on-metal design. Something better was needed, and Charnley's device looked to be a good starting point.

But there were significant problems with this pursuing this idea. The surgeons at Exeter had become accustomed to using a posterior approach to the surgery (i.e., through the back of the joint), whereas Charnley always insisted that purchasers of his prosthesis use a lateral (side) approach. The differences between the two techniques were not negligible.

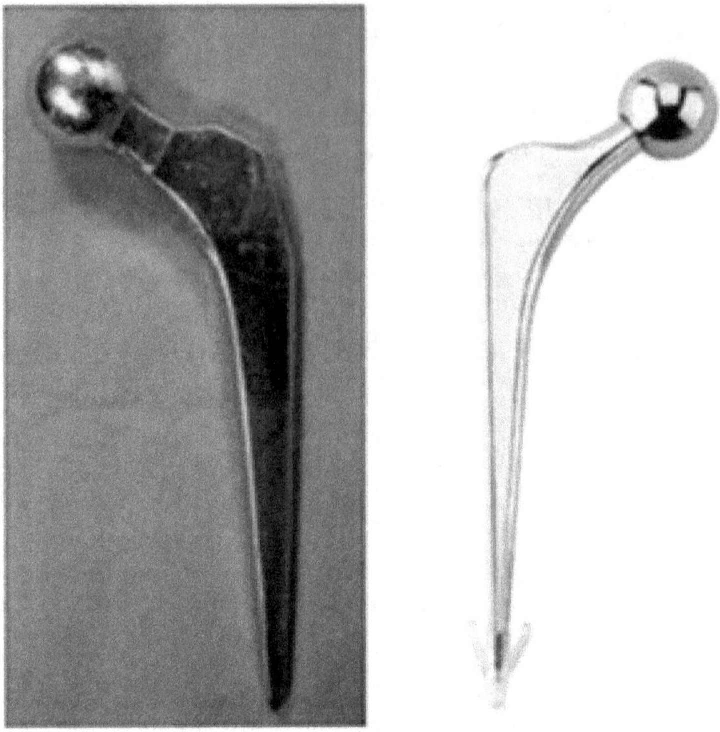

Exeter Hip / Source: Holy Cross Orthopedic Institute

To reach the bone, surgical incisions must safely traverse layers of tissue while avoiding major blood vessels and minimizing damage to other body tissue. Each path, of course, presents a different set of difficulties, which in turn require different surgical techniques. Adherents of each surgical model truly believe their chosen method is decidedly superior; hence a lasting disagreement over how best to access the hip socket. Ling and Lee were understandably unwilling to use what to them appeared to be the less desirable approach.

The Exeter team also faced a further obstacle if they intended to use Charnley's devices. Removal and reattachment of the femur's greater trochanter was an integral part of Charnley's procedure, but Exeter surgeons believed this carried an unacceptable risk of infection.

On the other hand, if they did not agree to follow Charnley in this regard, they would not be allowed to participate in the training at Wrightington or purchase prostheses from Thackray.

To resolve this dilemma the Exeter team ultimately chose to design their own prosthesis, one which differed substantially from other hip replacement devices. Their product would become known as the "Exeter Hip," which initially was sold exclusively through the London Splint Company.

The Exeter Hip used a metal-on-plastic prosthesis with cemented fixation and differed from other devices in two very obvious respects. One was the lack of a "collar" on the neck of the femoral component. This collar supposedly took much of the load and transferred it to the surface of the remaining femoral bone. Without such a collar, it was widely believed, the remaining bone would atrophy. However, the Exeter team had found otherwise when it reviewed follow-up X-rays of patients who had received McKee-Farrar hip implants, so they chose to omit the collar as unnecessary.

A second difference was the shape of the prosthetic stem inserted into the femur. Exeter used a "double-taper" stem, in which the stem itself forced the acrylic cement down into the femoral canal while it was being inserted, in order to improve fixation.

The Exeter Hip was first used in November 1970 after extensive laboratory testing. In a variation on Charnley's own restrictions on the sale of his devices, the London Splint Company agreed not to sell the Exeter devices to surgeons who had not been trained at Exeter until the group had completed at least five years of clinical trials.

Hard Choices

Complicating the search for the "best" hip replacement method for all the groups was a dilemma: the long-term consequences of using a given material or design might not become apparent for many years after the surgery. The same was true for fixation methods.

Yet conducting ten or fifteen years of clinical trials before going forward with a particular implant system was not a realistic option: the demand was too great. People were suffering, and the potential benefits for most patients far outweighed the risks. Moreover, the various implants seemed to be working well, and no law required surgeons or patients to wait.

The real question facing orthopedic surgeons was which particular mix of materials and fixation methods to use.

Making the Devices

Implant devices introduced in the 1960s and early 1970s reshaped not only the science of hip surgery but the business of orthopedic implants as well.

While the various British research groups were developing variations on or alternatives to Charnley's procedure, orthopedic manufacturers in Britain and the U.S. were beginning to compete for business in the rapidly growing total hip market. The usual first step was to negotiate an agreement with one of the research groups to manufacture a particular prosthetic device—obtaining such rights through acquisitions and mergers would be a later development—and a number of companies entered into such arrangements.

Thackray, of course, continued to manufacture Charnley's devices, while other manufacturers worked with the various researchers. But the field on which Richards Manufacturing competed was rapidly becoming crowded.

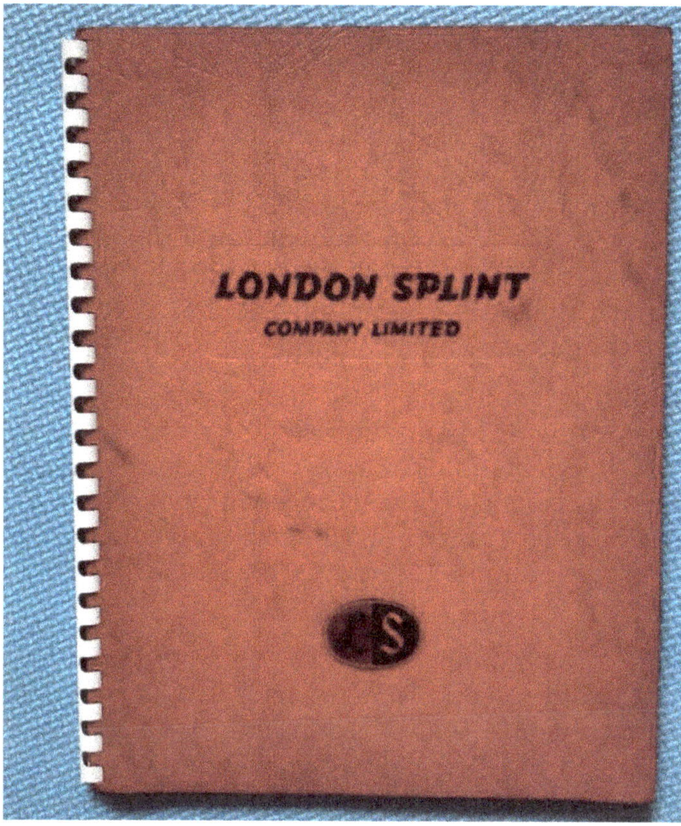

London Splint Company Catalog, circa 1958

Zimmer UK

An early and major competitor in the field, this one American-owned, had a familiar name—Zimmer. However, it was not Warsaw's Zimmer, not Zimmer USA, but Zimmer *UK*, and the difference was profound: Zimmer UK and Zimmer USA were entirely different companies.

Zimmer UK was the end product of a dispute that had its beginnings in 1938, when there was only one company with the Zimmer name. That was the year that Frank Saemann, who had been Zimmer's sales manager for six years, convinced company founder Justin Zimmer that a stronger European presence was needed if Zimmer Manufacturing was to compete on the international stage. It appears that Saemann and Zimmer were not in complete accord—to put it mildly—on how to do this, and Saemann soon found himself in virtual corporate exile in Europe. At any rate, Saemann moved to Europe and organized a new international sales force, but with some unusual contract provisions that left Saemann in effective control of European divisions that would eventually become Zimmer UK, Zimmer Holland, Zimmer France, etc.

Meanwhile, Zimmer's U.S. activities continued to operate under the name Zimmer USA. In the years that followed, Saemann did a remarkable job of marketing Zimmer products and, more importantly (especially to Saemann, as it turned out) spreading the Zimmer name throughout Europe.

However, when World War II broke out, a bitter dispute arose between Zimmer and Saemann, over profits and over the right to the Zimmer name. Because of soaring wartime demand for orthopedic products, name recognition and a great deal of money was at stake. The matter wound up in court and was not resolved until 1945, when Saemann prevailed.

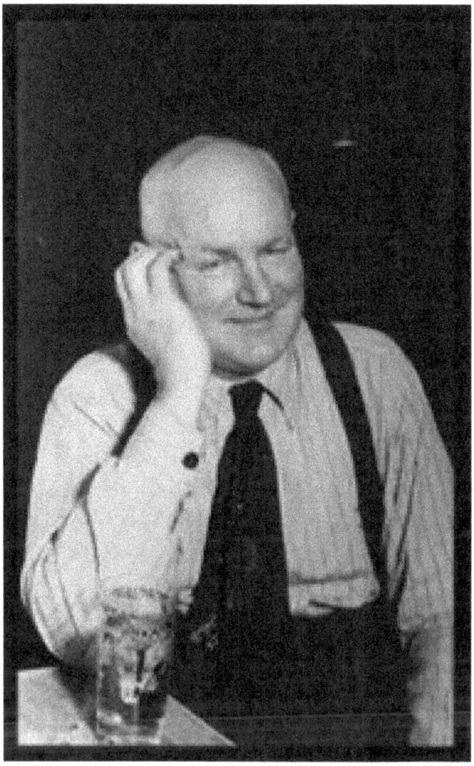

Franklin Saemann
Source: Saemann Foundation

Besides money damages, Saemann was given the right to register the name Zimmer UK (and other like-named European companies) and use the name Zimmer in marketing even though the true owner would be Saemann's new venture, the Orthopedic Equipment Company, or OEC. Saemann also apparently copied the Zimmer catalog page for page and reportedly even used Zimmer's catalog numbers modified only by a prefix or a suffix.

Not surprisingly, when Stanmore researchers needed a manufacturer for its new metal-on-metal devices, they turned to Zimmer UK, which was already a major player in the field. But despite the Zimmer name, Stanmore's agreement was actually with OEC. In fact, OEC would retain control of the Zimmer UK and its

European affiliates until 1982, when Zimmer USA's owners paid Saemann $14 million for the exclusive right to use the Zimmer name. Nor was Stanmore the only research group that would do business with Zimmer UK.

Down Brothers

Down Surgical was a home-grown British manufacturer that in the mid-19th Century had started out as a maker of medical instruments for surgeons at Guy's Hospital in London.

The company eventually came to be owned by Arthur W. Down and his brother Hubert, and as Down Brothers, Ltd., it earned a reputation as a manufacturer of quality surgical products. Business grew steadily and by 1951 Down Brothers had begun its own marketing operation for orthopaedic products made in both the Europe and the United States, including Stryker beds and a range of orthopaedic instruments. Its catalog that year also included both Judet and Smith-Petersen hip prostheses as well as modified Judet models.

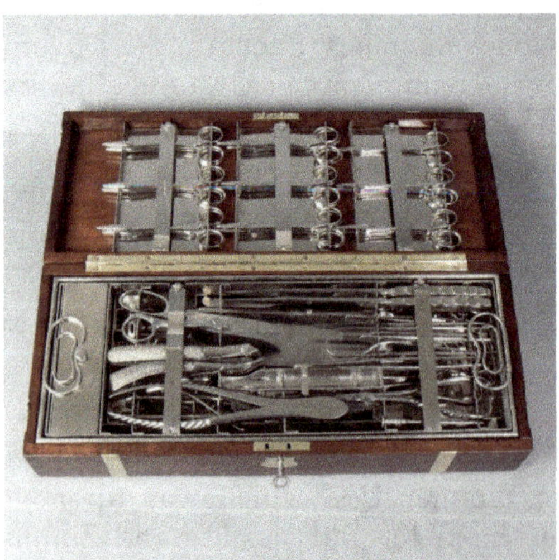

Down Brothers Instrument Tray circa 1960s

Source: Gerald Mathias

Soon the company was also marketing an even greater variety of orthopedic implants, including the Moore and Thompson femoral models. Down Brothers—it would become Down Surgical, Ltd., in 1972—was in fact the initial manufacturer of Redhill's total hip replacement prostheses, but this did not last for Ring eventually switched to Zimmer UK to make his devices.

Deloro Stellite

Another competitor to enter the total hip field, albeit somewhat later, was Deloro Stellite, a manufacturer of sophisticated alloys such as chrome-cobalt. The company had moved into instrument and device marketing in the 1950s, but it was not until 1972 that it established a branch company (Deloro Surgical Ltd.) to take advantage of the rising demand for total hip replacements and related surgical instruments.

Within a few years Deloro Surgical would be manufacturing several hip systems, all made from Deloro's own trademarked chrome-cobalt alloy called Vinertia and would do so for the rest of the decade.

Howmedica

Near the end of the 1960s yet another American company, Howmedica, acquired the rights to the popular Exeter Hip, although not through negotiations with the research group. Like Deloro Stellite, it was originally a metal manufacturer (Howe Sound) that supplied raw material to various orthopedic manufacturers, but in 1946 it had begun offering various implants made of Vitallium, a trademarked alloy of cobalt, chromium, and some other elements, and by the mid-1960s the company was specializing in chrome-cobalt products.

The company changed its name to Howmet in 1964, and four years later Howmedica was spun off as a separate company manufacturing orthopedic products. Almost immediately, Howmedica took over the London Splint Company and, consequently, production of the Exeter device, but its first years in this role were hardly auspicious.

Although the original design of the Exeter Hip had exhibited few problems, within two years of Howmedica's acquisition of the London Splint Company a number of broken femoral stems made it clear that a stronger stem was required. The breakages apparently were due to changes in the design of the stems that had been made by Howmedica for "reasons of symmetry and ease of manufacture." Pfizer would take control of the company in 1972, but problems with the Exeter Hip would continue.

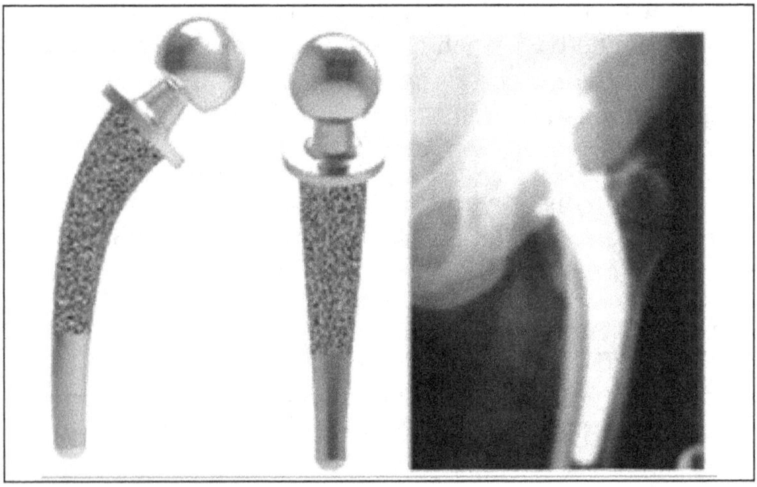

Biodynamics Hip by Howmedica / Source: Timothy McTighe

Zimmer USA

Back in Warsaw, Indiana, Zimmer USA was not sitting on its corporate hands and in fact had begun marketing its first hip prosthesis in 1950, a femoral-only implant it had developed in association with Dr. Palmer Eicher, working at the Indiana University Medical Center. This gave Zimmer USA an even wider product line, and by the end of the decade its sales were the largest in the industry. When the company received substantial backing from five wealthy local investors, the company was able to add even more products to its catalog.

During the same period, Zimmer USA also began experimenting with porous materials for its implants in an attempt to encourage biological fixation of the implants, and in 1971 the company would market its first Charnley-type system, using a metal femoral stem with a plastic acetabular cup. The following year Zimmer would merge with Bristol-Myers.

DePuy

What of DePuy, Zimmer USA's long-time Warsaw competitor? Its story was quite different, and it certainly was not as quick as other manufacturers to enter the orthopedic field. The company had grown steadily during the 1940s under the joint leadership of Winifred DePuy Leiter and her husband Herschel, and by 1950 it was the industry leader with more than fifty employees and some $3.2 million in annual sales. But a sequence of events led to a leveling off of the company business in the 1950s. Winifred Leiter died in 1949, and Herschel soon remarried, this time to Amrette Aile. When he died only a year later, she took over management of the company.

It was not a smooth transition. DePuy employees had been under the impression that Leiter had promised to leave the company to its salesmen, and an ownership battle took place. Amrette and her new husband—she married Harry Hoopes in 1951—prevailed, an outcome which would have a long-term effect on the company. Throughout the '50s and into the early '60s DePuy continued to record strong sales of its soft goods, but the company did not make any significant capital investments. In fact, its 1964 total sales were even lower than they had been in 1950.

Complacent is probably the best word to describe the DePuy top management at this time, and a 1956 article in the Warsaw *Times-Union* newspaper is unintentionally revealing: it describes a plant and manufacturing process that does not appear to have changed very much over the years. Although Mrs. Hoopes is portrayed as a hands-on manager, the article also mentions that she and her husband had been in Europe for three months the previous year. DePuy's top management seemed fully satisfied with what it had always made and sold.

This abruptly changed in 1965 when a group of investors purchased DePuy from the Hoopes family. J. Keaton Landis, who had been DePuy's sales manager, became company president and began to strengthen DePuy's market share by acquiring other companies and adding new product lines.

The turnaround was dramatic, and in 1968 DePuy secured exclusive marketing rights to the Müller Hip, a leading total hip replacement prosthesis. This expansionist approach was short-lived, however.

Also in 1968, soon after it purchased Kellogg Industries—another manufacturer of "soft" products such as braces and splints—DePuy was sold to Bio-Dynamics Corporation of Indianapolis, Indiana. DePuy Manufacturing now became DePuy Orthopaedics, and for the next five years Bio-Dynamics kept the company under close control and did not allow it to expand.

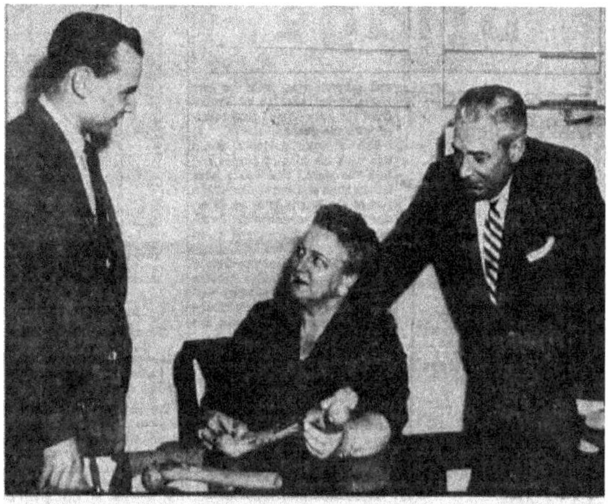

SALES TALK. — Mrs. Hoopes and her husband (right) and Keaton Landis, of Warsaw, sales manager for DePuy's, discuss business. Mr. Landis supervises sales representatives who cover the United States, Canada, South America and Europe. — (Times-Union Staff Photo.)

Mrs. Amrette Hoopes, DePuy President circa 1964
Source: yesteryear.clunette.com

DePuy's competitors, however, were not so hampered, and the industry experienced what can only be described as explosive growth in the late 1960s and early 1970s. But advances in hip replacement techniques and new prosthetic devices were not the only reasons for this. Another was a shift in how society looked at artificial joints: as more and more orthopaedic specialists came to see total hip replacement as a viable option for their patients, patients likewise grew accustomed to the idea as well. Replacing a section of bone with a surgically implanted prosthesis no longer sounded like science fiction.

And there was a further development in the 1960s that would have even greater consequences for the orthopaedic implant industry, especially in the U.S.

Halfway through the decade, a dramatic social policy change took place in America: the federal government, 20 years after President Harry Truman championed the concept of health insurance for the elderly, on July 30, 1965, at the Truman Library in Independence,

Missouri, President Lyndon B. Johnson signed Medicare into law.

Orthopedics Accelerates Dramatically and Richards New Team Finds Its Rhythm

By the mid-60s, Harry Treace had become Richard's driving force, working long hours and expecting others to do as much. His own technical knowledge and extensive engineering background in orthopedics enabled him to work closely with doctors to develop new products, and this was key to newer and better product development.

Ideas for devices and tools typically came from the orthopedic surgeons themselves, and engineers at Richard would then try to translate the surgeon's ideas into safe, effective, manufacturable, and salable products. It was a good system, but it had its limitations, as L.D. would recall:

"It was kind of a cumbersome process back then because we didn't have the computerized equipment that they have now. So, in a lot of cases, you had to build tools and dies to make products—which you couldn't do because it was too expensive."

Treace could also be impulsive, not necessarily a strength in what was becoming a tumultuous business environment. Fortunately, Bill Fisher, the CPA-attorney whom Treace had brought in as executive vice president to handle company finances, was fully familiar with the inner workings of Richards from his years as the corporation's auditor. He also became a member of the board of directors and in both roles was, in L.D.'s view, a much-needed stabilizing force in the company.

L.D. now 34-years-old, was in charge of all production, all personnel matters (including interviewing and hiring), and all purchasing for a plant that had nearly 80 employees and which annually produced several million dollars in sales. It was a position that also meant, as he and Betty had accepted as inevitable, even longer workdays, and the two of them soon settled on a pact. She would never call to remind him that dinner was ready, but neither would she hold dinner. "If he was not home by seven o'clock, I fed the children and put them to bed, and he came home when he could. He ate whenever he came in."

The major reason L.D. often ended up eating alone was that the title "plant manager" was somewhat misleading: his responsibilities were even wider, usually because Treace frequently gave him new projects to handle. For instance, in addition to dealing with salesmen and suppliers, overseeing production, and, as needed, resolving employee matters, it fell to L.D. to design packaging for every product that Richards made.

At the time, the packaging being used by Richards was barely adequate and did not look at all professional. When Treace brought this to L.D.'s attention, the message was clear. The plant manager took a hurried flight to Fort Smith, Arkansas, looked at a plant there to see it could make something that Richards could adapt, and rushed back to Memphis. L.D. would remember the trip as one that resulted in major changes in plant operations.

"It was sort of like somebody who's right on the verge of bankruptcy, and one more bill comes in and that throws him over the edge. That's the way my time was. [The Fort Smith trip] was that one more bill that came in, and I said I've got to get back and start delegating all of this."

"So, on the plane coming back, I just sat down and kind of worked out an organization chart. Who can I put in this? Do we have anybody in house that I can put into this job?"

This thinking quickly took him several steps beyond the problem of packaging: "Seeing salesmen—that's an all-day job because there's enough salesmen to keep you busy all day long. How do I set this up? So, I thought of somebody that I thought could do it. He was a recent college graduate who I thought could do it, and so we set up a purchasing department and put him in charge, and that worked out pretty well."

L.D. also decided that production control and personnel should be separate departments, and he penciled in the names of people he thought would be effective departmental supervisors. Upon returning to Memphis, he presented his ideas and his chart to Treace, who readily approved them, and L.D. was soon training the new department heads. He also resolved not to get bogged down in overseeing every decision the new supervisors made. For L.D., delegation would mean real delegation.

The trip and the reorganization had two other consequences. One was this new idea that L.D. now had time for other responsibilities that would pay long-term dividends (in this case, literally) for the company: "I could take on other things like looking at product acquisitions and company acquisitions and taking on some more responsibility in other areas once I got those things off my back and organized."

The second consequence, one L.D. may not have fully realized at the time, was a change in how he looked at his own role in the company. In the past, he had always willingly taken on responsibilities assigned to him by Treace, always looking for ways to improve a particular part of the company's operations. In that regard, the trip to Arkansas was typical: he was tasked to figure out a way to improve packaging. But now his thinking was going beyond his immediate assignment. How to make the entire operation better? How to improve product quality? How to stay on top of new developments? How to improve sales and profits? That would be his thinking from then on.

However, one task L.D. could not completely delegate was a special project Harry Treace entrusted to him in 1964: creation of a new product catalog.

For years, Richards' catalog of its orthopedic devices and tools was an ordinary plastic spine binder that included product information along with some rather poor black-and-white photographs of its product line. It did not convey the image that Treace desired, and over lunch one day he asked L.D. to come up with something better. Treace also needed it in time for the 1965 annual meeting of the American Academy of Orthopaedic Surgeons (AAOS). He wanted new photographs, new copy, and new artwork in a three-ring binder with a silkscreen cover. How hard could it be?

More than 30 years later, L.D. would still remember it as one of the most difficult assignments he ever undertook, although he was able to laugh about it: "I think that came as near to killing me as anything I ever did."

Product descriptions had to be technically exact, the photographs had to be sharp and clear, and the catalog as a whole had to present the company as modern and efficient—in other words, a company that a surgeon could depend on to produce quality products. The demands of producing the catalog meant another sharp learning curve for L.D., requiring him to meet with the printer on an almost daily basis. Although he had overall responsibility for the project, he would later credit others for the quality of the finished product. For artwork he relied heavily on the talents of Rick Mendius, a young artist who had joined Richards as a draftsman, and most of the photographs in the catalog were the work of Eli Jaffe, who ran a photography studio on Union Avenue.

"If I had any spare time during those early days," L.D. would recall, "I would be working on the catalog. I would go into town to Mr. Jaffe's studio and maybe spend the afternoon, or part of the afternoon—we'd lay out the photographs and do those."

L.D. also tried his hand at writing copy for the catalog, but it was painstaking, exacting work that he did not enjoy, and he would end up conferring with Treace about what he had drafted. In contrast, Treace had a genuine talent for composition, and he wrote or edited most of the written copy.

But L.D. did take some photographs that were included in the final version.

"I took the cover picture of the plant from the outside, and I had to take it at night with just the lights on in the building because it had so many overhead wires running to it that spoiled the picture. So, I got out there with a tripod and a camera one night and took pictures for the front of the catalog."

With the help of Mendius and Jaffe, and the cooperation of an understanding printer, the first copy of the new catalog was completed just in time for L.D. to take it to the AAOS 1965 annual meeting in Chicago.

The meeting was a new experience for L.D., who had not traveled much for the company, but Treace had insisted that he attend when the matter first come up:

"You are going to the Academy meeting, aren't you?"

When L.D. said he had not planned to do so, Treace simply said, "Well, you're going, and let's bring Betty, too." Don Richards would not have approved at all.

Attendees at the 1965 AAOS annual meeting were certainly aware of the new surgical methods being tried in Britain as well as the new designs for orthopedic devices. Both developments were revolutionizing orthopedic medicine. But the orthopedic surgeons and manufacturers in Chicago must also have been concerned about upcoming votes in the U.S. Congress, votes that might forever change the practice of orthopedic medicine. As it turned out, they were right to be concerned, for that is precisely what happened.

A few months after the AAOS meeting, a different kind of revolution would trigger an almost unbelievable expansion of the orthopedic industry. Implant surgeries would become almost commonplace, and this in turn would lead to even more rapid industry growth as well as significant improvements in the entire field of orthopedic surgery.

What brought about these changes was landmark federal legislation that signaled a seismic shift in U.S. public policy toward health care and how it was delivered and financed. In the summer of 1965, after a decades-long political battle, Congress created Medicare, a federal health insurance program *for the elderly* financed through mandatory contributions by employers and employees in the same manner as Social Security retirement and disability benefits. When the law went into effect the following year, some 19 million people—virtually every American over age 65—were enrolled.

Over time, more federal legislation and regulations would follow, each intended to protect patients and minimize risks associated with implant surgery. But Medicare was the turning point. The federal government had become an active agent in health care services, a role that profoundly affected not only patients and their surgeons, but manufacturers of orthopedic devices in particular. It probably should not have come as a surprise.

Medicare Becomes Rocket Fuel for Orthopedic Growth

Prior to 1965, the costs of medical care in the U.S. were borne by individuals and their insurance companies.

Although virtually all industrialized European nations had adopted versions of national health plans shortly after World War II, the U.S. had, in the main, continued and expanded an approach that had begun during the war years.

Throughout the war, employers had faced serious manpower shortages, and wage restrictions authorized by Congress in the Stabilization Act of 1942 meant that companies could not offer increased salaries as an inducement to prospective employees. A frequent solution to this dilemma was to expand fringe benefits—which were not subject to wage controls—especially medical insurance offered through employee group insurance plans. Both employers and employees benefitted: an employer could offer additional, relatively low-cost fringe benefits as part of its total compensation package, and the employee would not have to pay income tax on those benefits. Moreover, because group rates were based on the company's pool of employees, premiums were *significantly* less that premiums purchased by individuals.

This approach worked quite well for employees whose companies offered health insurance benefit, but millions remained uninsured—employees of small companies unable or unwilling to pay even reduced premiums, the self-employed, and, of course, those individuals who, for whatever reason, did not have regular jobs. Moreover, connecting health insurance coverage to employment also meant that coverage ended upon retirement (except for those individuals whose former employers provided health coverage as part of their retirement plans). This created obvious problems for older retirees. Insurance premiums for senior citizens were costly if in fact the retiree could even find a company willing to insure him or her. This was because older persons faced health care costs that were typically three times that experienced by younger persons.

How to address the healthcare needs of the elderly became a major social issue in the post-war years, both in terms of practicality and as a political issue. The central question became whether the federal government should become involved in what had always been a matter left up to individuals (or, as in most cases, the employers who actually selected the group insurance plans) and their physicians and hospitals.

Not that this was the first time the issue had arisen. It had first come up when Social Security was enacted in 1935, and it was the subject of intense debate in the 1940s, when a series of proposals were considered by different Congresses. Each was opposed by the American Medical Association, and none made it to the floor of either house. Hearings were held on several bills in the late 1950s, but only one—to expand state-run welfare programs to include "medical indigency"—made it into law. New efforts during the Kennedy Administration were likewise unsuccessful; sometimes opponents felt that a specific proposal went too far, while counterproposals, such as one supported by the AMA, were opposed because they did not go far enough.

The political dynamics were different in 1965 when President Johnson was sworn in after a landside electoral win that also brought strong Democratic Party majorities in the Senate and the House of Representatives. Again, there was strong opposition from the AMA, through its lobbying arm AMPAC, but public sentiment and demographics were changing. The elderly population had grown from 12 million in 1950 to 17.5 million in 1963, and the cost of hospital care was rising at a rate many times that of the cost of living.

The battle in Congress was passionate, but the ultimate issue—whether there was to be some form of national health care for the elderly—was probably not in doubt once several powerful Democratic members of

Congress, including Congressman Wilbur Mills, chairman of the House Ways and Means Committee, endorsed the idea. The real issue was the form that the new law would take.

What emerged were the now familiar—at least to older Americans—Medicare Parts A and B: the former covered part of the costs of hospital care, and the latter dealt with outpatient services, including physician's fees and testing. If a person paid into the system, he or she was covered upon reaching age 65 (or even earlier if certain disability requirements were met). In short, the U.S. government became the nation's largest health insurer. And because it was set up as a government-run insurance program financed by a new payroll tax on employers and employees, eligibility was not based on need.

At the same time, Congress also created Medicaid (Title XIX of the Social Security Act), a program which provided health care to the needy. It was funded jointly by the federal government and the individual states, but, unlike Medicare, it was administered by the states, and eligibility was based on an individual's income and assets. A further difference was that Medicaid coverage was not limited to the elderly and disabled, so many welfare recipients were also included.

Although the cost of Medicaid would eventually become a major item in the federal budget, Medicaid expenditures for orthopedic implant surgery would remain only a tiny fraction of that paid by Medicare and private insurance companies. According to a study conducted four decades after the two programs were created, Medicare was paying for roughly 58% of all total joint replacement procedures, about ten times the number of such procedures covered by Medicaid. The rest was paid for by private insurance companies or by patients themselves.

The impact of Medicare (and, to a much lesser degree, Medicaid) on the orthopedic industry was unforeseen.

but when it did, it transformed the practice of orthopedics. Like the American Medical Association, orthopedic manufacturers had uniformly opposed Medicare, and the leadership at Richards Manufacturing was no exception. They saw it not only as socialized medicine, undesirable in itself, but also as the first step toward government control of the industry. No one, it seemed, gave much thought to the possible economic impact on the industry.

But it turned out that there was a significant upside to the new law, not only for patients, but for surgeons and orthopedic manufacturers as well. For the first time, a large group of potential patients (the elderly) who often needed specific medical services (in this case, hip, and knee implants) now had a third-party payer (Medicare) to shoulder the cost. Prior to the advent of Medicare, many older Americans needing a hip or knee implant in order to walk safely without pain simply could not afford the surgery. Now, with the advent of Medicare, they could.

There was also another factor. A major social phenomenon, already begun but barely perceptible at first, coincided with the growth of orthopedic implants. It, too, would have a significant impact on the rising demand for orthopedic implant surgery.

Earlier generations had typically viewed joint pain and varying degrees of disability as part and parcel of the aging process: human body parts simply wore out, and people adjusted as best they could with the aid of glasses, hearing aids, canes, and walkers. But as older Americans began to realize that disability was not necessarily destiny, the demand for medical implants to reverse otherwise disabling conditions soared.

Richards, like all the other orthopedic implant manufacturers, was totally unprepared for what happened next, as L.D. would later acknowledge:

"I don't think we had really calculated the effect of Medicare on making it available to everyone that wanted it or needed it. What I noticed almost immediately, just with a few months, was that these little hospitals around Mississippi and Arkansas and so forth, that used to buy a $16.50 Jewett nail to pin a hip, were now buying a $75 hip prosthesis just to replace the whole ball right into the socket."

"It was not a complete total hip. It was just half a total hip it replaced. It went down in the femur and replaced the ball of the hip, and that's what they were doing. It caused us all kinds of inventory problems after that happened, and the reason they were using it was because it was paid for."

The consequences at Richards were significant. In a very short time, the new 37,000 square feet Brooks Road plant—the one that was to last for years, maybe forever—was as squeezed for space as the previous location had been. And because the new building was intended to be permanent, even the office walls had been constructed of concrete. What had once looked so big to L.D. was now clearly inadequate:

"In a couple of years, we began knocking out walls. The first wall we knocked out was for a little break room we had. We took that in for these employees who were finishing the [Shea stapes] and packaging them."

But that helped only a little, and further stop-gap measures were adopted. A metal building was erected behind the original structure, and the company frequently had to rent additional warehouse space. By 1966, Richards had to build a major addition to the original facility.

Treace believed in rewarding people who worked hard and produced results, and he saw to it that the L.D. received appropriate and tangible rewards for a job well done. But as always, he was close-mouthed about his intentions. The car was the first signal.

At the time of the plant relocation, L.D. still owned a 1962 Plymouth, which he routinely used when he would pick up visiting surgeons at the airport. The problem, he told Treace one day, was that his car had no air conditioning—a distinct disadvantage in Memphis during the summer months—and that he was going to have one installed. But Treace had a better plan:

"No. Don't do that. Just go to Charles Reed and lease you a Buick. The company will pay for it."

In fact, Treace liked the idea so much that he told L.D. to also lease new cars for Smitty and for Calvin Griggs, the shop superintendent. This was somewhat overwhelming for L.D., who was used to Don Richards' well-known frugality, but he hardly had time to notice:

"That was quite a learning year for me. Things were moving so fast; I don't think I really had time to think very much of it. Just go where I had to be, day in and day out. Just do it and get it done."

And this was not the end of it, as L.D. soon found out.

In those days, the Beards were living in a very modest neighborhood in Southhaven, Mississippi, just across the state line, which suited them fine, but Treace would repeatedly tell L.D. that their home was, well, not good enough. L.D. always dismissed the suggestion, saying that he would get around to moving, probably to Whitehaven, in south Memphis, when he could afford it. He was not asking for a raise—he was simply telling Treace, in a nice way, that he was not concerned about it and that Treace should not be concerned either. L.D. was clearing about $200 a week, and he felt they were living quite well indeed.

Again, as with the mystery office, Treace was coy when he came into the plant one Saturday and told L.D. that he had increased his salary. L.D. did not ask how much it was, but he later decided to find out from the bookkeeper. It was a whopping 30% raise, more than enough to finance a new home. Betty found one she liked in Whitehaven, not far from the office, and the Beards moved in.

Another pay increase later that year made it possible for L.D. to buy some stock in the company. Dal Beard's son—who had taken a genuine risk when he had left a good job at Firestone and who had dropped out of college with little more than trust in a new mentor—finally had something to show for his labors. And there was still a lot of work to do.

CHAPTER SIX: NAPKIN DRAWINGS, INNOVATION, MEMPHIS, MANUFACTURING, WARSAW

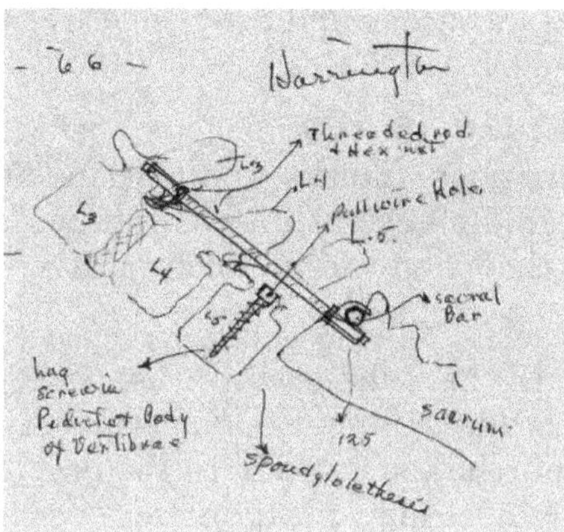

Paul Harrington's Sketches for his pedicle lag screw invention: circa 1966

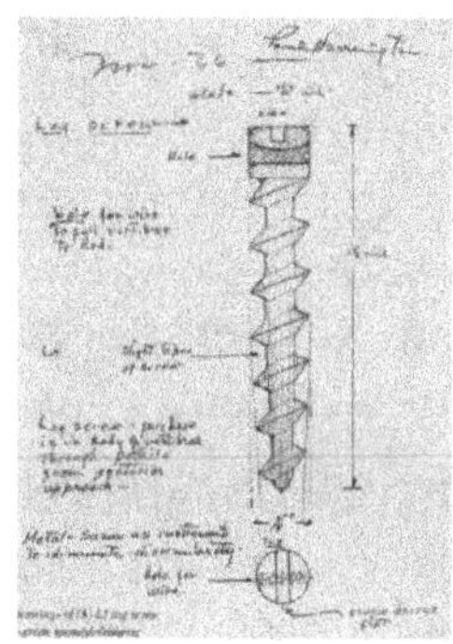

Today, the business of supplying orthopedic and spine instruments, implants and biologic products is a multi-billion global industry—which is dominated by U.S. based companies—Zimmer (Warsaw), DePuy (Warsaw), Stryker (Kalamazoo), Medtronic (Memphis), Smith & Nephew (Memphis), MicroPort (Memphis).

How a technology that was originally developed in the UK, France, and Germany, would come to be dominated by U.S. based companies is testimony to the innovative capabilities in Europe and the business and logistics acumen in the United States.

At Richards, Treace was the initial force behind expansion into international markets, and Canada. Sales were growing rapidly and cash flows even more so. Treace believed that an international presence would be worth the investment. L.D. fully agreed.

Both Treace and L.D. had discovered that many Canadians, like Americans, had a strong nationalistic bent when it came to purchases. Put simply, there were real advantages in having a maple leaf on the cover of one's catalog.

But Treace and L.D. wanted even more: "We wanted an office presence there with a Canadian manager, a Canadian corporation that would also be able to do inspection, packaging, and so forth, of products that we might send up there."

The first step was to establish relationships with Canadian banks, and both men flew to Toronto in January to scout possible locations, a visit that L. D. would long remember: "The Canadian Imperial Bank of Commerce had arranged for a limo and driver for us, because we were doing business with them, to go around and look at all these sites. You'd look at one of the warehouse sites where they had the back-up for the truck, but you couldn't tell where the back-up was because it was covered with snow. I finally said, let's just pick a place and decide that's going to be good enough, and go home. It was so cold and miserable."

This suited Treace, and after their return to Memphis Treace placed L.D. in charge of starting up the new Canadian subsidiary, which became Richards Surgical, Limited. Toronto was chosen because it would allow the company to reach potential buyers in both the English-speaking and French-speaking population centers. The Toronto plant initially did light manufacturing—rib belts, arm slings, and the like—and also served as the main sales office, although company sales representatives were scattered throughout the country.

L.D. also discovered that sales in Canada were conducted differently than in the U.S.: "The selling part of it was done mostly to the major medical centers. They sort of controlled a whole lot more of the market than the in the U.S. We sold mostly to major hospitals, major institutions. And it wasn't nearly as spread out and diversified with individual doctors' offices as you would see in the U.S."

Another difference was the vastness of the country, which posed difficulties for salesmen trying to reach someone in New Brunswick or one of the other provinces. Travel from Toronto to Vancouver was a major undertaking.

Because of these and other differences, such as customs issues related to imports, the Canada subsidiary would become a model for how L.D. would later conduct business in other countries: "They knew the regulations and they knew what they had to do, and they operated more or less autonomously from the U.S. operation. We tried to develop financial statements that were meaningful by bringing information in, but as far as operating the company we offered a great deal of autonomy to the managers."

Treace's aggressive leadership, together with Fisher's business acumen and L.D.'s organizational skills, paid off in terms of business growth: between 1964 and 1967, net sales at Richards nearly doubled, from $1,867,942 to $3,643,818. Corporate profits were also respectable, but the chief goal was to continue growing the company even larger and stronger. This was not ego or self-aggrandizement on Treace's part; it was just good business sense.

He was certainly aware of the slump that DePuy had fallen into. In the 1950s DePuy had failed to build upon its early success. Now, with so many new devices being developed and so many companies entering the market in the 1960s, solid growth was more important than ever. And if this goal was to be met, more cash would be needed.

L.D. believed that the company might have been able to generate the necessary cash, but only if it had sharply reduced expenses, and this Treace was unwilling to do. His inflexibility on this point did not please Fisher—L.D. would later say that it "caused Bill to pull his hair out"—but Treace held firm. Then, in 1968, Treace believed he had found a way that would help advance his plans without cutting expenses: sell the company to a bigger, well-established corporation.

The company's board of directors now consisted of Treace, Fisher, and L.D.—who had replaced John Stivers following his death in 1967—but it was still Treace's company and his call.

At the time, the leading firm in the area of corporate acquisitions was W.T. Grimm & Co. in Chicago, and Treace worked with them to find a suitable buyer. However, the process was not as quick as Treace wanted, and he soon grew impatient. Decades later, L.D. would describe what happened next:

"Bill was a one-man show, and Harry had talked to him. We'd have several people down, kind of kicking the tires, but nothing of any consequence."

"He finally went into Bill Grimm one day and said, 'Don't send anybody down just to look. If you've got someone interested in paying five million dollars for the company—our annual sales were close to four and a quarter million dollars or something like that—'we'll sell.'"

Rorer

In the early years of the 20th century, William H. Rorer had founded the pharmaceutical business that still bears the family name. It made and sold a variety of products, but its most notable success occurred in the 1950s, when it began to market the liquid antacid Maalox. By the late 1960s, Maalox accounted for 85% of Rorer sales, and the company began looking for investment opportunities.

Soon after Treace gave Grimm a specific figure, Gordon Moyer, Rorer's chief financial officer, came down to look over Richards' operations. He was soon followed by John Eckman, Rorer's CEO.

L.D. thought that the $5 million asking price was too low, and he was later convinced he was right: "You know when you've sold too cheap because [Eckman] came down and talked around it, and finally said, 'Well, let's get to the real thing. How much do you want for the company?'"

Harry replied that the price was five million, and Eckman instantly agreed.

The purchase of Richards Manufacturing and its Canadian subsidiary by Rorer—the first acquisition of a major orthopedic company by a larger corporation—was completed in early June of 1968. The new company became the Rorer Group, Inc., and Treace remained president of Richards, now a subsidiary corporation. He apparently assumed that everything would remain the way it always had been, but that was not to be.

New Owners, New Products, and a Diffusion of Focus

Richards was not the only orthopedic manufacturer undergoing a change in ownership. 1968 was also the year that Bio-Dynamics bought DePuy, and a year later Howmedica purchased the London Splint Company. In addition, the ink was barely dry on the new stock certificates when two pharmaceutical giants decided to follow Rorer's lead and enter the orthopedic market with purchases of their own. In 1972, Pfizer bought Howmedica, and Bristol-Myers acquired Zimmer USA, quickly adding several smaller, medically related companies to make and market products under the Zimmer name. Rorer had been the first pharmaceutical company to enter the orthopedic implant business—now there were three.

Such mergers typically served the needs of both parties. Because new orthopedic devices were entering the market at a bewildering pace, manufacturers of those products often needed funds to expand operations in order to keep up with the competition. Moreover, if a manufacturer was fortunate enough to develop or acquire its own high-demand device, the need for investment cash was even greater. At the same time, some larger corporations were, to put it bluntly, cash-rich and needing to invest some of their earnings into other likely ventures.

It was much the same with Rorer's acquisition of Richards, for Rorer's investment enabled Richards to continue its mind-boggling growth. Part of this was surely due to increased demand for established products, much of it traceable to Medicare coverage, but another part of this and later growth was directly attributable to new devices—those designed by Treace himself or brought into the company by him—and to significant product improvements.

In both cases, having the necessary technology was essential, and the management at Richards was quick to realize that often the most advanced manufacturing technology could be found in the burgeoning aerospace industry, much of which was located in California. By the mid-1960s Richards already had a successful distributorship in the state—the West Coast was a major market for its products—and following the death of the distributorship's manager Richards opened a large shipping warehouse near Los Angeles. It would not be the company's only California connection.

Because of Richards' experience in manufacturing Dr. Shea's stapes, it was logical that the company would be alert to new developments in the field of otology. At the time, an increasingly popular treatment for chronic ear pain and infections in children was to place "vent tubes" (called "drain tubes" in the 1960s) in a child's ear to help fluid drain out, and Richards took the early lead in this market. But there was a problem.

The technology used by Richards produced the tubes one at a time on a lathe, a very slow process, and the company was soon overwhelmed with back orders. L.D., the plant manager, became concerned about this bottleneck but was told by the shop superintendent, Calvin Griggs, that there was no other option. L.D. thought, otherwise, and he was soon on his way to Los Angeles with schematics and samples. He chose Los Angeles both because of the company's presence there and because it was home to myriad aerospace and plastic machining companies. When he arrived, however, he had no idea which of the many aerospace companies in the area would be able to help him—there were several listed in the local Yellow Pages—but good fortune took him to a manufacturer in El Segundo:

"The first one I went to was a place called Royal Industries, and I went in and talked to the president. I told him what I wanted and needed. I said, 'Now, they're going to be coming from an outside source.

They've got to be public. No shortcuts or anything like that. They've got to look just like what we're making.'"

The company president assured him that his facility could handle it, but he was curious about the size of the order L.D. was talking about.

L.D. decided to ask for about a year's supply, around 38,000.

No problem, said the president.

This left only one issue, the one that had brought L.D. there in the first place: how long would it take to manufacture that many devices? The answer astonished him.

"Oh, you'll get them in two weeks."

L.D. could hardly believe that a full year's production could be completed in just 14 days. Yet when he returned two weeks later and examined the tubes, he could detect no difference in appearance or quality. All 38,000 tubes fit into a small package, and L.D. was so pleased that he was tempted to take them with him on the plane. But he thought better of it. What if the airline lost his luggage? He figured no one would believe how valuable the package was. The tubes were shipped and arrived safely, and Richards was able to catch up on its back orders.

Hips, Knees and So Much More

A very different product, one that was to have a much greater impact, would take L.D. back to California: Richards was about to introduce its first total hip replacement system.

Zimmer USA was already into marketing its own metal-plastic hip implant, but its device was a German import, and DePuy was still struggling under the Bio-Dynamics yoke. Moreover, neither Stryker nor Howmedica had produced a successful total hip prosthesis. This created an opening for any American company willing to enter the field, and Treace was determined that Richards would capture its share of the market. In fact, as L.D. later recalled, Treace had worked on his own prosthetic design but had not been successful:

"We'd been trying to come up with something for several years. Harry Treace had experimented with, and we had actually done, a couple of them using Teflon. Just the regular hip prosthesis in Teflon, and that didn't work. The Teflon would shave off and create problems in the hip joints. There was no way, no good way, to keep the Teflon part in the acetabulum. Everyone in the business knew that some way or another there had to be a way to replace the entire hip because that's what actually went bad, especially with arthritis."

John Charnley's success with his low friction arthroplasty in the UK had changed everything, and it so happened that one of Treace's surgeon friends had worked with Charnley early on.

Dr. Charles Bechtol, a professor of orthopedic surgery at UCLA, had been one of the first American physicians to perform a Charnley-style hip replacement, and he had immediately recognized that the surgical instruments used in the procedure needed modifications if the surgery was to be successful in the U.S. This was due to differences in how American and European doctors typically performed surgery: American surgeons wanted to be "in and out" as quickly as was safely possible in order to reduce the chance of infection, and the instruments being used in the UK and Germany actually slowed down the operation.

To deal with this problem, Bechtol designed surgical instruments that would facilitate a faster procedure, and Treace was eager to fabricate and market the instruments as well as the implants. The only downside was that Richards did not yet have the level of technology needed to micro-finish the heads of the femoral stems. Extreme smoothness of his prosthesis was essential if Bechtol's system was to work.

L.D. did not yet know the solution, but he knew someone who might. He called his friend at Royal Industries, who pointed him in the right direction. Royal Industries could not make the device, but its president knew of a company that had exactly the technology L.D. was looking for: a machine shop in Santa Monica.

The owner of J.C. Clark Company had recently died, but the previous owner, Elwood Phillips, was continuing to manage the company temporarily as a favor to Mr. Clark's widow. He told L.D. that the shop could do the work Richards needed, and the two men reached an agreement.

As promised, the finished products fully met Richards' specifications, and L.D. quickly saw advantages in buying the Clark company outright: the shop manager was anxious to leave the business and also wanted the owner's widow to get some money out of it. Basically, Richards could have the company for the value of its machinery and equipment. And there was an added benefit: the company's experienced employees were willing to remain at their jobs. L.D. felt it was too good a deal to pass up, and he presented the proposal to Rorer management. He would later laugh at their response:

"They wanted to know about what [the assets] would be worth, and just from walking through it I estimated $175,000. And they said, 'We'll send an appraiser out there and we'll see.'"

"They hired an appraiser and sent him out, and he counted everything, including the wastebaskets I think, and he came up with $176,050." L.D.' s aptitude tests at Whitehaven High School had not been a fluke.

This apparently satisfied Rorer, the sale went through, and Richards no longer had to contract out its micro-finishing.

The Bechtol Hip was virtually the same as the Charnley device, and it was an instant success when Richards introduced it in 1970. As the first cemented hip manufactured in the U.S., it would soon account for 30% of the total U.S. hip market. It probably helped that company representatives regularly attended courses on total hip replacement that Dr. Bechtol conducted for orthopedic surgeons at the Hollywood Roosevelt hotel.

L.D. also became friends with the doctor and through him witnessed a major difference in how UK and U.S. doctors viewed hip replacement. In the U.S., any patient, young or old, in overall good health or not, could be the recipient of a total hip prosthesis. Not so in Britain, where surgeons restricted the surgery to patients who were considered good candidates—i.e., in good health otherwise and not truly aged—for a successful surgical implant. The feeling among British doctors was that the surgery should be reserved for those most likely to benefit from the procedure. A real-life example of this difference in attitude and philosophy would remain with L.D. long after he left Richards:

"I remember Dr. Bechtol called Dr. Charnley at one point and said, 'I have a patient. She's seventy-some-odd years old. She's obese. What would you use for her surgery?'"

"[Charnley] said, 'Don't use anything. She's a poor choice.'"

Richards' new California operation would soon undergo a major expansion. Harry Treace's son James and his friend Barry Bays, another Richards' employee, submitted a proposal for the two of them to run the plant. L.D. and Harry Treace reviewed the proposal, both liked it, and L.D. persuaded Phillips—who was still running the plan on a temporary basis—to stay on until they became familiar with plant operations.

James had already demonstrated that he had inherited his father's skills in developing new products—L.D. knew him to be "one of the best products developers in the business"—and Bays was experienced in manufacturing the actual devices. They made a good team.

James Treace had joined Richards soon after college, and Bays had been brought in by L.D., albeit by a circuitous route. When L.D. was studying aircraft maintenance at Whitehaven High School, the "shop" program there was run by a man known to everyone as "Doc" Fisher, and L.D. had developed a great respect for his talents. Not long after L.D. became plant manager, Fisher had called L.D. to recommend a student for employment. The young man was about to graduate and was, according to Fisher, "the most talented student he had ever had."

L.D. was more than willing to give Bays a chance, but there was a slight problem. He knew that Griggs, Richards' own talented shop superintendent, would not take kindly to someone in management hiring a shop employee. On the other hand, if Bays was as good as Fisher had said, L.D. did not want to risk losing him. So, he devised a stratagem.

L.D. went ahead and hired Bays to work in the plant's inspection department, and within a couple of weeks Griggs came in to tell him about a phone call he had received from Fisher, whom Griggs also knew:

"Doc Fisher was telling me about a kid he had in the machine shop who was the best he had ever seen. We need to see how we can work around and get him in the company."

When he told L.D. the young man's name, L.D. innocently said, "Calvin, he's on the Richards payroll and working in Inspection. You can put him in the machining shop any time you want to."

Bays did, of course, work out, as did his joint project with James Treace in California. After their arrival in Los Angeles, the J.C. Clark Company became Richards Surgical Manufacturing Company—RSMC for short—and became, in L.D.'s words, "our primary producer and, with the help of Harry, our primary designer of total joint implants."

Something was clearly working right. By 1968, the year Rorer acquired Richards, Richards' net sales had climbed to nearly $4.7 million, and in 1970 the figure reached $8 million. Two years later, the number was just under $12 million, and in 1973 the company's net sales would pass the $15 million mark.

The Modular Knee Innovation

Not long after the Bechtol Hip came onto the market, another California doctor began an important, but ultimately unhappy, relationship with Richards Manufacturing and Treace.

Although not as well-known as Dr. Bechtol, Dr. Leonard Marmor was also a pioneer in orthopaedic surgery, but his key work focused on another joint—the knee. He had held a variety of medical teaching positions in the Los Angeles area and in 1969 joined the staff at Saint John's Hospital in Santa Monica.

It was while Dr. Marmor was at Saint John's that he and Treace got together—L.D. was also at the meeting—and developed a new knee implant system based on Marmor's ideas. The new implants were to be modular in design, meaning that the surgeon could choose which parts of the knee to replace and which to leave intact, and Treace showed him how the components could be manufactured and used. This was important because the damage might be to a femoral condyle—the anatomical term for a rounded prominence at the end of a bone, especially where it interacts with another bone—or, in some cases, to more than one condyle. A modular system allowed the surgeon to customize the prosthesis to suit a patient's individual needs.

Of course, having so many replacement options in one joint meant that each component had to have the same level of polishing and smoothness as the micro-finishing of the femoral head in a total hip replacement. Fortunately, Richards now had the necessary tools to do this—the machining equipment that L.D. had been instrumental in acquiring for Richards had become a major asset—and the Marmor Modular Knee, complete with micro-finish, could be produced in quantity.

After Treace and Marmor worked out a licensing arrangement, Marmor submitted a patent application for the new prosthesis in early 1973, and Richards began production of the device. As with the Bechtol hip, the response was immediate and positive:

"Once we developed this product with Dr. Marmor, it took off and we were back-ordered heavily. Everybody wanted it. We showed it at the Academy meeting [the American Academy of Orthopaedic Surgeons]. There was no FDA approval back then, so if you had an idea, you produced a product, then you showed it, and you sold it."

Other companies soon copied the modular design, which did not surprise L.D. "Our competition got into it very quickly. We did have it patented, but they kind of built around the patent because it was such a revolutionary new product."

Comfort Care

Notwithstanding the new focus on the manufacture of artificial joints and the external frame, Richards had continued to manufacture and sell its soft goods products, and in 1969 the company had relocated its sewing department to Pontotoc, Mississippi, a small town about two hours' drive from Memphis. Three years later, at about the same time that Richards was developing the Marmor prosthesis, the company took a further step and decided to spin off this entire soft goods line into a new subsidiary there.

The idea had arisen out of discussions between L.D. and Bill Fisher, Richards' executive vice president. Both men believed that while the company's sales personnel were neglecting these products—an understandable neglect, perhaps, given the expansion of the orthopedic implant side of the business—and that a small company making quality soft goods could be highly successful. They saw a potentially large market for such items through contracts with hospitals and surgical supply dealers, both of which could stock the products in quantity.

The plan was for the new company, called Comfort Care Products, Inc., to take over all of Richards' soft goods production, and they presented the proposal to Rorer. The parent company approved it, L.D. was named Comfort Care's president, and he was scheduled to assume management of the operation on April 1, 1973. But there was an unexpected delay to a personal mishap.

When L.D. was a boy, his family had considered him accident-prone:

"When I was almost seven years old, I was riding my bicycle as fast as I could, going from one side of the road to the other, and hit some loose gravel. I was unconscious for three or four hours. One of the neighbors brought me home, and I'm sure my mother about had a heart attack. Then, a year or two after that, I broke my leg at school, and she got a call that I was in the hospital."

L.D. was reminded of the "accident-prone" label thirty-odd years later when, the day before he was to arrive in

Pontotoc, he climbed a ladder in order to saw off a tree limb:

"I sawed the limb off right even with the tree, and it was a big limb. When the end hit the ground, it came back up on the ladder and started to push me over backwards. The tree was too huge to try to hang onto, and I didn't have a limb to hang onto or anything else, so rather than just fall backwards, I jumped off the ladder."

He tried to clear the concrete sidewalk, but did not, and his heel bones and back were broken. Betty witnessed his fall, which must have frightened her, but her nursing training paid off:

"I guess I went into the nurse mode because the first thing I remember doing was—he had on paratrooper boots—to take those off. I think I got Tylenol or aspirin, and I brought the car around to the front of the house."

"At first, I wanted to call an ambulance because I was afraid of a back injury, but he was insistent that we weren't going to call the ambulance. We were going to go in the car. He could get in the car if I would bring it to the front of the house, so I did. He did manage to get into the car—which we should never have done, because he did have the back injury."

After arriving at Methodist South Hospital in Whitehaven, they took X-rays that prompted the X-ray technician to observe—L.D. found this ironic—"Boy, are you ever going to need a bone doctor!"

Fortunately, the back injury was a compression fracture, which usually mends itself over time. He was hospitalized for nearly two weeks, had casts on both legs for six weeks, and had to wear a spinal brace for at least six months. In August, when he had recovered sufficiently, he and Betty finally moved their family to Oxford, Mississippi, a university town about thirty miles west of Pontotoc.

Comfort Care was a much smaller company than Richards—in terms of personnel it was about the same size that Richards had been in 1960—but in the nearly two and a half years that L.D. was Comfort Care's president the subsidiary's workforce roughly doubled in size to meet demand. However, the company was not the unqualified success that L.D. and Fisher had hoped for. Richards' sales distributors remained less interested in selling conventional soft goods than other products manufactured by Richards, especially its popular orthopedic implants. This attitude hampered sales and frustrated L.D.

Nor was Comfort Care the only demand on his time and attention. Mindful of his acumen in pushing the J.C. Clark Company acquisition, Rorer increasingly called on L.D. to evaluate other potential ventures, and Richards—meaning Treace and Fisher—still relied upon him for assistance. Although he now lived in Mississippi, L.D. routinely had to spend a day or two each week at the Richards office in Memphis.

The reason was L.D.'s unmatched familiarity with plant operations there, which continued to encounter snags because demand for Richards' devices had become so heavy that the current Brooks Road facility was simply inadequate. As a temporary measure, the company even moved its sales and marketing department to leased space in an office park near the Interstate, but communication between the department and the plant suffered as a result. The answer was to erect a new building at the old site.

The plan was to house all manufacturing in a new 65,000 square foot building behind the current facility and convert the existing structure—which had already undergone several expansions beyond its original 36,000 square feet—into office space and shipping. The problem was that Eric Clarke, who had been head of facilities management in Memphis and who would have been the logical person to oversee the expansion, had been sent to Los Angeles to manage a new subsidiary and did not wish to return to Memphis.

He asked L.D. if he would do it, and L.D. said he would. Or, to be precise, L.D. said that he would except for one thing: that Richards already had someone in the Memphis plant who could do the better than he could.

"Who's that?" Fisher asked.

CHAPTER SEVEN: RON PICKARD: THE MOST CONSEQUENTIAL MANAGER OF THEM ALL

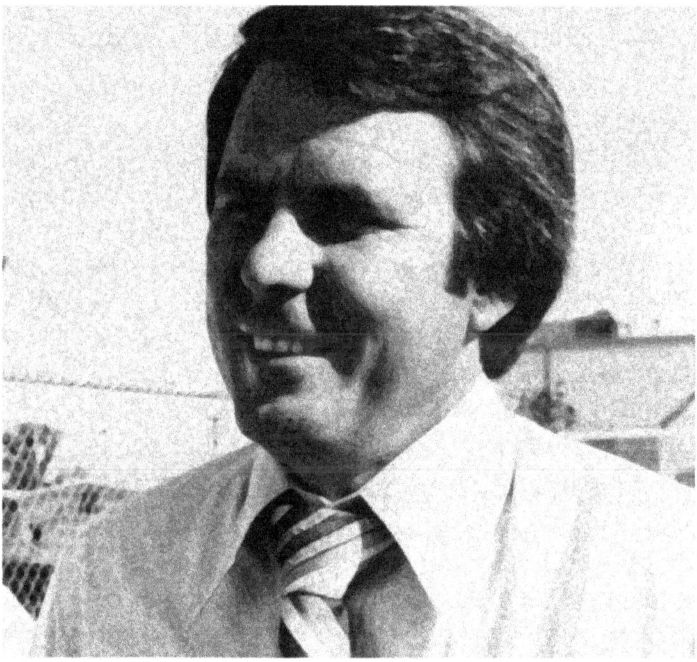

Ron Pickard, President of Richards Orthopedics, circa 1979

In later years, L.D. would laugh when recounting how Pickard would say that he had known L.D. since 1967 but that L.D. had known him only since 1972. Which, L.D. would admit, had some truth in it. Pickard had made his way up the Richards ladder much as L.D. himself had a decade earlier, although starting at an even lower rung. L.D. had joined Richards as a shipping clerk; Pickard's first job there was janitor. But even though the latter was 16 years younger—Pickard was born in 1948 in Tipton County, a few miles north of Memphis—the similarities between the two men reached even further back.

L.D.'s grandparents had been tenant farmers, and Pickard's grandfather had been a sharecropper, although those distinctions often blurred. Like L.D., Ron learned about hard work at an early age, chopping and picking cotton and working in cornfields from daybreak to dark to earn money to buy clothes for school. And at age thirteen, he also learned about initiative, buying a lawn mower on credit at a local hardware store so he could earn additional money mowing yards along the highway.

Also, like L.D., Pickard developed a genuine respect for his schoolteachers, realizing that they truly cared about the students. More than four decades later he would recall how during his senior year his English teacher had made sure that he graduated; it was not tutoring in the usual sense but sitting down with him every day after school to make sure he understood the importance of studying. Work was important, but so was self-discipline.

Pickard married his high school sweetheart shortly after graduating high school and found a job at the RCA factory in Memphis—it paid $1.85 an hour—but he quickly decided it was not what he wanted. After only two weeks, he quit and began looking for better opportunities in Memphis, there being no industry in

Tipton County at the time. And then he more or less stumbled onto Richards Manufacturing.

It was 1966 and 19-year-old Ron Pickard was in his 1966 VW Beetle (which he'd purchased new for $1,700 plus tax and was paying $49 on the monthly note) driving down Brooks Road in the industrial park near Memphis's airport looking for work.

Pickard and his new wife, both graduates of Munford High School, were still living in Munford, about 34 miles north of Memphis in Tipton County—named, incidentally, after Captain Jacob Tipton, who was killed while leading a charge of his troops against a force of Indians in 1791 near Fort Wayne, Indiana.

Munford, Tennessee (population 100, on a busy day), originally Mt. Zion, was in the rich. loamy Mississippi River delta where settlers from North Carolina, Virginia, Kentucky, Alabama, and Eastern Tennessee had come in the 1830s.

"I had graduated from High School. I had but two pennies in my pocket and I needed a job." Pickard remembers. "I was driving down the road, saw a sign out front of this building that said "Hiring", pulled in and it happened to be Richards."

Don Richards had been gone for three years, the company was booking about $3.6 million in sales, growing 25% annually and Harry Treace and L.D. Beard ran the company.

Pickard put in his application.

"There was a lady at the front desk. I will never forget her. Miss Alma Fife. I walked in and told her I wanted to apply for a job, and she was a really nice lady. She directed me all the way back, and there was this guy sitting with a metal cage all around him with all these supplies. A tool room type of thing. He was sitting there doing paperwork and I stood there and stood there and stood there."

The man was J.W. Torrey, who supervised maintenance at the plant, but he did not introduce himself.

Pickard finally asked if he was in the right place.

"Yep," he was told, but it was several minutes before the man said anything else:

"Do you see that big die up there on the top shelf?" he asked.

"Yes, sir," said Pickard.

"Do you think you could get that down and clean it and put it back?"

"Yes, sir."

"Go on up there, and she'll tell you when you start."

That was the interview. He was soon working upwards of sixty hours a week, sweeping floors, and doing other custodial jobs:

"When I wasn't doing that, I cut metal. They had these big, long rods of stainless steel that would have to be cut into certain lengths to go out to the machine shop for certain parts to be made, so with an abrasive saw I would cut the rods to a certain length."

And he especially liked the work atmosphere at Richards.

"Quite honestly, I didn't know enough to know whether it was a big company or a small company. It was a company. And I'm coming fresh off the farm. I knew it wasn't as big as RCA—at least the building wasn't—but other than that I really didn't give much thought one way or another whether it was large or medium or small. But it was one of those situations where no matter what you were doing—whether you were sweeping the floor or running errands or cutting metal—you were a part of Richards. You know, you weren't something less than somebody else. It was a good atmosphere."

1967, the Pickard became the 84th employee of Richards, the Scoliosis Research Society (John Moe, President) had wrapped up its first year. Paul Harrington, Professor of Orthopedic Surgery at Houston's Baylor College of Medicine, had sketched out the concept of a lag screw to be used in the pedicles of the spine, performed two spondylolisthesis cases with the screws and written a paper about it, which was presented in 1967 at the Southern Medical Association's 61st annual meeting.

In England, Sir John Charnley's new hip prosthesis and reconstruction surgical procedure had demonstrated that hip replacement surgery was viable, reproducible and could, for the first time, give elderly and arthritic patients sustainable pain relief and a return to a functional life.

In Switzerland, Maurice Edmond Müller, M.D., professor at the University of Bern and head of orthopedic surgery at the Inselspital in Bern founded Protek AG, to manufacture and market the Charnley-Müller hip prostheses. Müller was also one of the principal founders of the AO Foundation.

Pretty much the only spinal implant on the market was Zimmer Corporation's (Warsaw, Indiana) Harrington Rod.

In Memphis, the Campbell Clinic dominated regional orthopedic care and was among the top five orthopedic teaching hospitals in the United States. It's founder, Willis C. Campbell, M.D., was the first president of the American Academy of Orthopaedic Surgeons. No coincidence, Richards Manufacturing's first location was directly across the street from the Campbell Clinic.

Just outside of Memphis, Frank Wright, a former Richards Manufacturing salesperson, had started Wright Medical to fabricate and sell a rubber walking heel for patients in leg casts. At the time, patients in leg casts were complaining of chronic back pain due to the hard steel heel built into the foot of their casts.

Pickard was joining Richards just as the orthopedic and spine industry was hitting its legendary growth spurt.

Ron and his wife Linda continued to live in Tipton County, and the trip to and from work took about an hour each way. Pickard never minded the drive, but it became more difficult once he moved up to the polishing department, which occurred after he had been there a couple of years. To hear Pickard tell it, the offer came out of the blue.

Pete Porch, who had been with Richards since its early days, supervised the polishing department and approached him directly: "I've got this position that will pay you a little more than what you're making now, if you want to come over here."

Torrey, Pickard's supervisor in maintenance, was not happy with the transfer, but for Pickard it was an opportunity to get into the business side of plant operations, and he would end up working in the polishing department for five years. But the advancement came at a price: Pickard had to arrive by 5:00 a.m. every morning to turn on the boiler an hour before the rest of the employees arrived, which meant he had to leave home at four o'clock.

Soon, Porch was telling L.D. Beard about the fine work that Pickard was doing. As L.D. later recalled, Porch had "never before come up to me and talked about employees like that. He'd stop by my office and talk, but he had never done that."

And then there had been the matter of the Dale Carnegie course. L.D. felt that he had benefitted from the course during his early years at Richards, and he now made sure that all departmental supervisors enrolled at company expense. He did this not to turn them into public speakers but because, in his words, "I wanted them to be able to deal with people."

Pickard heard about this practice and enrolled on his own. When Porch mentioned this, L.D. was impressed: he knew that Pickard did not make that much money. Pickard was someone to keep an eye on.

Later, when Fisher asked L.D. whom he had in mind to supervise plant maintenance and oversee the new plant expansion, L.D. had no doubts whatsoever:

"When I told Bill that Ron could do it better than I could, he was kind of in disbelief, so he said, 'Well, let's take him to lunch.'"

They took him to the University Club, one of the oldest and finest private clubs in Memphis, hardly the kind of dining that Pickard was used to. L.D. would later comment that it was probably the first time Pickard had even been to a private club, and Pickard jokingly added that it also the first time he'd ever used a cloth napkin. True or untrue, the business they discussed over lunch was serious, and Fisher was impressed with the young man and gave him the job.

Pickard had been in his new position only two or three weeks when Fisher took L.D. aside: "That's the smartest little devil I've ever run into. He just turned that job upside down. Did you know he was that smart?"

Leaving Comfort Care

Although L.D. was able to solve Fisher's immediate problem without returning to Memphis, other demands on his time, both from Richards and from Rorer, together with three other troubling factors, were giving him pause. He was beginning to think that it just might be the right time consider other opportunities. Perhaps start his own company.

One of the factors causing L.D. to examine other options was that Richards Manufacturing had changed: it was not merely much, much larger than the company L.D. had joined in 1960—it was *different*. More politicized somehow. The second was that Treace's two sons—understandably, in L.D.'s view—were now in key company positions and were being groomed for further advancement. L.D. felt this was natural, and he wanted to avoid any possible conflicts.

Finally, there was an unexpected problem with the modular knee, a problem that would wind up in court—actually, in more than one court—and have repercussions for years. Some of the facts remain in dispute, but what is clear is that there was an early manufacturing error in one component of the prosthesis: due to an engineering error, one artificial condyle was slightly larger than it should have been. The error was discovered, and steps were taken to correct the problem, but not before the wrong-sized implants had been used in a number of surgeries. Some patients experienced serious consequences, resulting in litigation based on claims of malpractice and products liability law.

Because Richards had a sizeable inventory of the larger condyles, it wanted to keep them in stock and clearly label them a different size. But what the company did not take into account was how Dr. Marmor would react to this. He believed that the licensing agreement between him and Richards specifically required his approval of any changes to the components. Neither side was willing to budge, arguments ensued, and tempers flared.

The patent for the knee prosthesis was issued in December 1974, and two days later Dr. Marmor announced he was repudiating his agreement with Richards. Lawsuits followed—including one by Marmor for libel—and L.D. was glad not to be directly involved. Yet he was, as he would later say, "watching from the sidelines," and it was always the main topic of conversation whenever he visited Treace and others in the Memphis office.

This was understandable. When the problem with the knee component was discovered, Harry Treace's son James had met with Dr. Marmor to try to resolve the problem, but the meeting had become acrimonious, and the relationship between Treace family members and Dr. Marmor soured. During each visit to the Memphis plant, L.D. would be acutely aware of the tense atmosphere there.

And yet, despite all the controversy and rancor, Richards' sales growth continued apace. The same year that it began producing Marmor's modular knee, Richards' net sales reached $15.2 million, dwarfing all previous sales figures. The following year, 1974, the figure would be just under $21 million, an increase of nearly 38% in one year. Other manufacturers were enjoying similar success.

Leaders within the orthopedic industry were aware of the role that L.D. had played in the success of Richards and its subsidiaries, and he was beginning to receive job offers as well as offers to help him go into business on his own. Also, despite the less than enthusiastic promotion of soft goods by Richards' sales force, Comfort Care was performing well, and L.D. felt that he had accomplished about all he could there. L.D. decided it was indeed a good time to move on.

At some point in 1975, he shared his thoughts with Fisher, telling him in strict confidence that he was "thinking about looking into trying to buy into another company and getting some equity someplace and be able to run my own show. I said I don't know if I want to start from scratch or not because that's kind of hard to do, but I think there are opportunities out there."

This evoked a surprising disclosure from Fisher: "Before you decide to do that, I want to tell you something I haven't told anybody else. I'm going to go on partial retirement the first of the year. I haven't announced it yet. Harry doesn't know it yet. Nobody knows it yet, but I'm going to go on partial retirement for a year and then I'm gonna fully retire. I'd like to see you get my job."

And then he made one last pitch to bring L.D. back to Memphis. Would he consider returning to Memphis as a vice president? It would also be a return to a previous title: when Rorer had acquired Richards, L.D.'s responsibilities had remained much the same, but he had been given a new title: Vice President of Operations.

This way, as Fisher presented his idea, when Fisher fully retired, L.D. would be the likely choice for executive vice president. Said Fisher, "I'd like to see you get my job." L.D. genuinely regretted Fisher's decision to retire—they had been through a lot together—but Fisher's mind was made up, and L.D. agreed to accept his offer. In December 1975 he returned to Memphis as a vice president of Richards Manufacturing. This time L.D.'s position was simply vice president, but when the occasion demanded a more exact title, he would use "Vice President, Corporate Development."

Fisher had not told anyone else of his retirement plans, much less the part about L.D. taking his place when he did retire, but L.D.'s return to Memphis went smoothly, nonetheless. Because of his frequent visits to the main office, he was hardly a stranger. And despite the ongoing conflict over the Marmor Knee—or perhaps because of it—Harry Treace certainly seemed happy to have him back. In some ways it was as if L.D. had never left.

It turned out to be a timely return, for both the industry and Richards itself were about to undergo another round of major challenges and changes.

Pickard Moves Up the Ranks

Pickard had quickly adapted to his new responsibilities as head of facilities management, and he especially enjoyed working on the new building project. It was the kind of challenge that he enjoyed, and it also brought him into frequent contact with L.D. upon his return to the Memphis plant. Although Pickard was deeply involved in coordinating the construction of the new manufacturing facility, it made sense for L.D., who had handled a similar project when the Brooks Road plant was built, to oversee the project. But L.D.'s role in this move was more often supportive rather than directive. As for Pickard, he was glad for the opportunity to work directly with someone with L.D.'s experience, and he gladly accepted his leadership.

The two men worked well together, and their relationship reflected L.D.'s managerial style. Whenever he became aware of an employee who displayed initiative and talent, L.D. would find a way to give that employee a new task with new responsibility, much in the same way that Treace had done with him. His new title was a bit vague, but titles had never been that important to L.D. For him, what counted was furthering the company's interests, and this often meant dealing with the matter at hand. And in Pickard, as L.D. had suspected, he found a like-minded person. Under L.D.'s direction, Pickard was given responsibility both for planning the new addition and for the extensive remodeling of the old facility.

For Pickard, the experience was downright fun: "What I think I enjoyed the most about it was the ability to have a little bit more of the planning side of it as opposed to just the execution side of it. Now you not only had to get something done, but you had to determine what needed to be done."

"One of the first things L.D. had me to do was determine what type of space and how much space are we going to need. So, we went about actually analyzing every department—how much activity was going on and the flow of product from one department to another. You could go into the break room and sit down and have a 30-minute discussion with a supervisor about the work going on in his department and pretty well get a good insight. I didn't particularly think one way or the other about quote-unquote 'supervising people.'"

"We got everybody involved in it. We had little team groups that were going to be responsible for moving every piece of equipment. We moved the whole thing on the weekend."

This was followed by the gutting the old building, and Pickard would always remember the day L.D. showed up to inspect the work:

"We hired a bunch of day laborers with sledgehammers, and we just started demolishing the inside of the old building. L.D. walked out one day, and he looked, and it was a mess. There was a cinder block lying in the middle of the floor, and wires were hanging from the ceiling. He looked at me, and he said, 'I sure hope you know what you're doing.'"

He did, of course, as L.D. already knew. Over time, the two men would have even more interaction, and Pickard believed he had found the secret—or at least one secret—of L.D.'s success:

"Working for L.D. is unique, in that you don't have to be worried about whether or not you're trying to please *him*. It's the job you do. And that means not only getting the job done, but how you get it done. Do you work well with other people? Do you get it done through other people or with other people? And you don't have to be scared of failure. You know that he's trustworthy. You know that he's as good as his word, and if you exercise good judgment and you've done the best you can, and you fail, that's okay."

"I've never been exposed to anyone like L.D. that could handle the upward focus in an effective manner [while] his real interest, his real concern, was downward in the organization—where things were happening. He realized that people like myself were paying their house notes, buying a car, and paying a note on that car based on his job. And so that made a big impression."

CHAPTER EIGHT: THE ILLIZAROV EXTERNAL FRAME

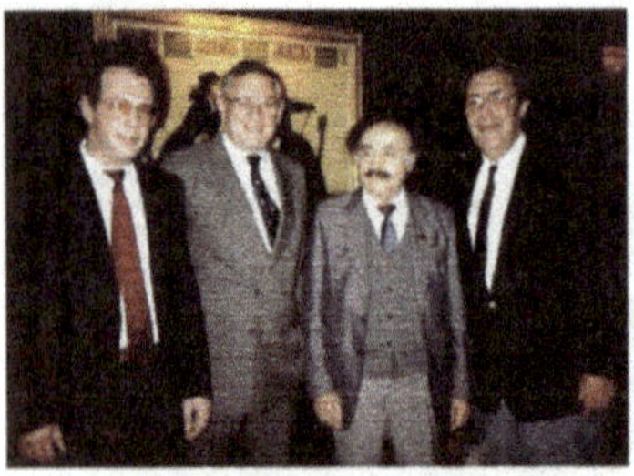

Victor Frankel with Ilizarov. On the far left is Michael Samchukov who travelled with Ilizarov and then immigrated to the US and works at Texas Scottish Rite in Dallas. On the far right is Al Grant, also one of the first adopters of the Ilizarov method who worked at the Hospital for Joint Diseases with Victor. Ilizarov regularly visited with Victor Frankel in New York during his US trips. Victor even arranged for him to undergo emergency vascular surgery in New York.

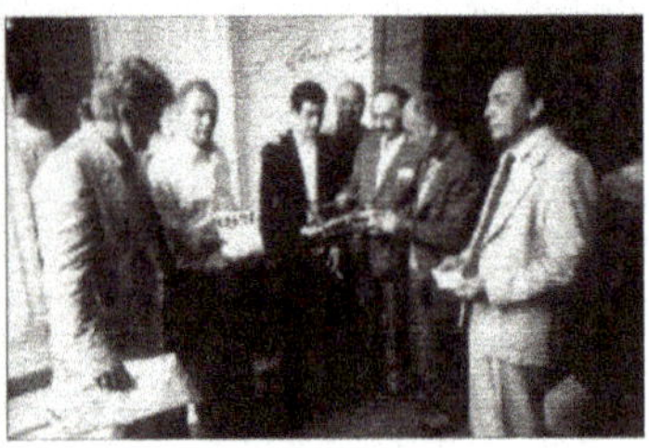

Professor Ilizarov demonstrating his external fixator to a group of surrounding physicians. His signature is on the photo.

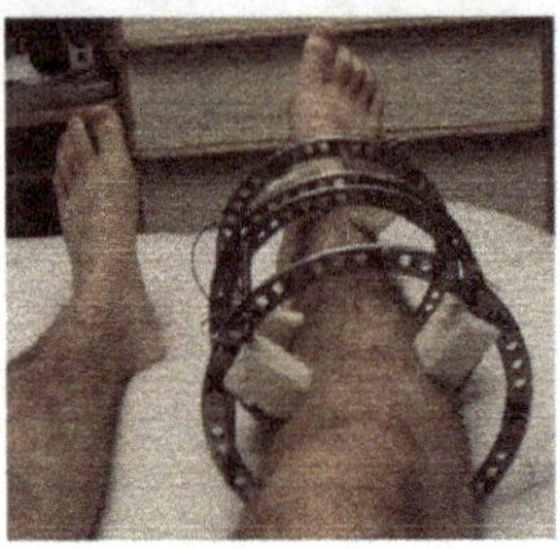

An Ilizarov apparatus treating a fractured tibia and fibula of the lower right leg

Around the time that L.D. first met Don Richards in the lobby of the company that bore his name, on the other side of the world, in Siberia, a young physician was trying to find a way to heal non-union fractures. He came up with a true first-of-its-kind approach—a metal frame made from bicycle parts which connected directly onto the patient's skeleton through the skin.

With this frame holding the bones in a fixed position, this physician, Gavriil Abramovich Illizarov, could precisely cut the bone, distract it by a couple centimeters and induce bone's natural healing mechanism and close the manmade gap with new bone. Twenty years would roll by before word of the Ilizarov extraction method frame reached the Western medical world.

And when it did, it generated an orthopedic earthquake.

Rick Treharne, who was the first Ph.D. employed at Richards, was head of R&D and one of his research projects was the artificial ligament. In 1984 he hired a young man with experience in artificial ligaments from Meadox Medical in New Jersey, Alex Lukianov, to be an R&D manager. Meadox had developed a Dacron-based artificial ligament for the shoulder and anterior cruciate ligament (ACL).

The story behind the Illizarov frame begins with a famous adventure book and movie, *Kon Tiki*. A book that really stuck in Dr. Treharne's mind.

"One of the books I read in High School was *Kon Tiki*, where the famous adventurer Thor Heyerdahl sailed a handmade boat from Mexico to the Polynesian Islands," recalls Treharne, "They did a follow up version of that called *The Ra*, where they took the same type of boat from Egypt and tried to get to America."

"They had this international crew leaving from Egypt. "Ra" is the Egyptian word for 'Sun' and 'Ra' is the Aztec word for Sun. They thought there was a connection there. On this international crew was one guy who was Russian, one guy was Italian, Thor Heyerdahl was Norwegian. The guy from Italy was Carlo Mauri. Carlo Mauri had a non-union in the tibia which was putting out pus all the time. He was a venturesome guy, so he was going across the Atlantic Ocean. The crew had a lot of time to get to know each other and this guy from Russia asked about Carlo's tibia."

"Carlo says 'my doctor has been trying to fix it for years and can't fix it, doesn't work...'"

"So, the Russian doctor, Yuri Senevich says, 'If we live through this, why don't you come see me in Russia, I know a doctor here who can fix anything.'"

"After they landed, Carlo Mauri, who was very famous in Italy for his explorations, went to Russia with his mate from the ship and goes to see this doctor in Siberia named Ilizarov."

On April 4, 1980, Professor Illizarov operated on Mauri. He distracted Mauri's nonunion by 2 cm, healing the pseudarthrosis, correcting the equinus deformity by distraction, and lengthening his leg.

"Mauri's Italian doctor, when he saw what Illizarov had done, his eyes just about fell out of his head," recalls Treharne, "Ilizarov, who'd been working pretty much in obscurity in Siberia had hundreds of patients he'd treated. One guy, an amputee, Ilizarov grew his bone out, then turned it at a right angle to make a foot. Miracles. That was he called them. Walking miracles."

"Carlo Mauri's doctor, Dr. Bianchi-Maiocchi from Milan, was so shocked by what he'd seen—he'd tried six times and failed to cure Mauri's non-union. So, Mauri's doctor went to Siberia to see Ilizarov. In Siberia, they were making the spokes of the frame out of bicycle parts."

"Dr. Bianchi-Maiocchi had his son start a company to make the Ilizarov frame for him in Italy. They did and they made it better with stainless steel wires and frames and everything fit together well. Dr. Victor Frankl in New York went to a meeting and heard him talk about this and told Jack Blair, who was president of Richards at the time."

Blair assigned the Ilizarov project to Rick Treharne.

"Jack Blair and I flew to Switzerland and had a meeting with Dr. Bianchi-Maiocchi and cut a deal to see if we could bring this to the United States. That was an adventure. The doctor we worked with in Canada was Dror Paley and he was the guy who actually made it happen. He'd heard about Ilizarov too. Paley is an amazing guy—speaks Russian, French, Hebrew, and could probably figure out Spanish and French in his spare time. He wanted to bring it to the West too."

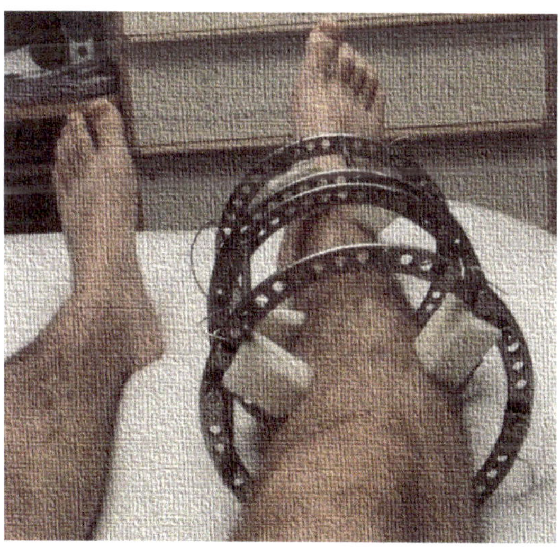

Illizarov External Frame in Use

Dr. Dror Paley

Dr. Dror Paley of Toronto, Canada, then a fourth year orthopaedic resident at the University of Toronto, heard about the Ilizarov method in November 1983 from Dr. Renato Bombelli, a world-renowned hip surgeon who was a Guest Professor of the Annual Rehabilitation Conference.

Paley had presented a case of a tibial bone defect and Bombelli told Paley that in Italy, they would treat such a case with the Ilizarov method in which bone would be shifted gradually from one end of the defect to the other. Paley had no idea what he was talking about. He quietly asked Bombelli about this during the coffee break. Bombelli drew a diagram to explain.

Paley realized that no one in the room had understood what Bombelli was talking about either but had been too polite or embarrassed to ask. Paley wrote Bombelli asking for literature on the subject, while at the same time, he performed a literature search. All he could find was Russian language references on the Ilizarov method.

Paley was surprised to find an enormous body of scientific literature on Ilizarov, even though as far as he could tell no one had ever heard of him. Paley connected again to Bombelli at the 1984 American Academy of Orthopaedic Surgeons (AAOS) meeting. Bombelli gave Paley Italian literature on the Ilizarov method which stimulated him to visit the Italian centers at the end of his residency in 1985.

That same year Paley presented two papers at the Richards Orthopedics Resident Conference and won first prize for both and was awarded $10,000 for research for each paper by the President of Richards, Jack Blair.

Paley was 30 years old, and he put Bianchi-Maiocchi in contact with Jack Blair from Richards. This began the negotiation and relationship between Bianchi-Maiocchi's Italian company, Medical-Plastic, and Richards, which remains until this day under Richard's purchaser, London-based Smith and Nephew. Paley refused to accept any payment, consulting relationship, or royalty from Richards or Medical Plastic for brokering this deal.

He was, however, funded by Richards Manufacturing to perform a biomechanics research project on the Ilizarov apparatus, comparing it to other fixators. Jack Blair also made a trip to Lecco, Italy to see the device with Victor Frankel. Blair also arranged for Paley to also visit Frankel in July 1985.

The Illizarov External Fixator Project Accelerates

The Illizarov project was percolating along, not the highest priority, at Richards when, unexpectedly, a telex from Licenintorg, the department of the Russian government that handled licensing matters, arrived in Memphis.

"We received a telex from the central governmental body out of Moscow that did all licensing deals." remembers Lukianov, "It kind of came out of the blue. Rick Treharne, who was head of research, said 'hey, don't we have some guy downstairs that we hired that can maybe speak Russian? Let's see if he can read it.' So, they brought the Russian License proposal down to me and said, 'can you read this?'"

"I translated it for them and, ended up, the Russian guys were reaching out to see if Richards would enter into a discussion around the Illizarov fixator technology. One thing led to another and two, three months later, I was on an airplane with Jack Blair flying to Siberia to meet with Illizarov for the first time."

"At Richards in those days a lot of us did things for the first time. Nobody showed you how to do things or gave you a template to follow. There were no instructions. So, I was figuring this Illizarov thing out on the fly."

"Putting together educational courses, it turned out, really set the pace and the tone for everything. Frankly, it was like the AO model that Synthes had advanced. If there was anything to emulate it was their AO model. I was always fascinated by that. Look at the kind of brand loyalty Synthes generated because of AO, who were all Synthes customers."

"We set up a similar model with Illizarov Method courses. What's really interesting to me about all of that was it was also kind of a marketing ruse. Everybody assumed that we did a deal with Illizarov, but we never actually closed a deal him."

"We did everything we could to close one. But it never happened for a variety of reasons including Gorbachev's "Perestroika", which allowed institutions to enter into agreements directly with Western companies. But there was a problem. They did not have a clue on how to go about negotiating a transaction!"

"What ended up happening was we (Richards, then owned by Smith & Nephew) went ahead and trademarked the Illizarov name. The man himself never did. So, for us, we were like, 'wait a second, this guy never trademarked his own name?"

"So, we trademarked his name, the symbol, everything. Everyone thought that the 'Original Illizarov from Richards' that we had branded was a license deal and that we had the technology. In fact, we had no protection around the Illizarov technology outside of Russia whatsoever. Inside Russia the Illizarov intellectual property wasn't really enforceable. So, there was no intellectual property outside of the Illizarov name."

"I was sent over to Russia multiple times to try to do a license deal. And ultimately they all fell apart."

"Illizarov didn't trust anybody. The guy was a very interesting character and appropriately paranoid living in the Communist system. For example, in his hospital, his entire 300 surgeon hospital, he personally carried the key for the Xerox machine in his pocket. Nobody was allowed to make photocopies without his permission."

"Ultimately, the relationship between Richards and Professor Illizarov became more about paying for educational programs in Russia and around the world. We simply paid for his time and to this institute to train other surgeons."

"With Dr. Paley, the Italians, Victor Frankel we put together an educational framework that ultimately led to a foundation and a series of associations, which still exist today with a reasonably sizable membership. The first one was in New York."

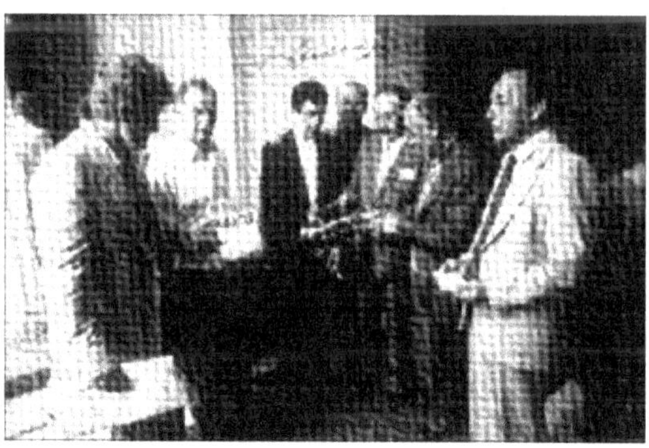

The Illizarov External Fixator Project

"I will never forget that I convinced Rick Treharne that we needed to hand out ties with the Ilizarov logo (as the surgeon societies do for AAOS, NASS and so forth). At the first course, we made around 150 ties, hoping for 75 or so participants plus faculty would actually show up."

"The production quality of the ties was not very good. Some of the logos did not reproduce well on the tie fabric. I started to sort them out and throw the bad ties into the garbage."

"In the meantime, however, we were overrun by attendees and the ties with the Ilizarov logo were being grabbed like hot cakes. I was busy running the course, negotiating, unpacking, dining, and doing it all, so I didn't have time to sift through all the ties at one sitting. I could only do it in batches."

"Each time I would sift through a batch of ties, I would load up the garbage can and then get distracted only to come back to an EMPTY garbage can."

"This went on several times before I realized that the surgeons were going through the trash to get a tie. That is when I knew that this Ilizarov fixation system could get big, really big, as I liked to say."

Bridging the Cultural Divide Between Russia, Illizarov, and America's Ortho Entrepreneurs

Alex Lukianov, now a legend in his own right, had the amazing fortune to cut his teeth on what would become Orthopedics' first viral orthopedic device—the Illizarov External Fixator.

As Treharne remembers, "It was an orthopedic earthquake back then. Everybody wanted it. It was interesting to me. The doctors said 'you only need to have the best doctors do this'...everybody was telling me that...because they thought they were the best doctors. It just took off, like a rocket."

For Lukianov, however, it was a crash course in cross-cultural medical training and license negotiations.

For example, Illizarov claimed that he never had a complication. Not a single one. Which, Lukianov remembers to this day. “Well, the big thing when doing the Illizarov method was to preserve the periosteum as much as possible and cut the bone in such a way that you did not compromise blood supply to the bone. The Ilizarov method was to advance a millimeter a day and perform a quarter turn four times a day. And it worked.”

“What would happen is that some surgeons expected a complication free process.”

“Illizarov’s mentality was different. In his mind, what is the complication? He really only thinks about terminal outcomes. Doesn't mean the patient won’t have some swelling, infection, or other issues along the way. To Illizarov, it was, all about, how does the procedure ultimately end?”

“He would get up at the podium and tell the surgeons ‘I have no complications’ and they're thinking ‘that's impossible’. Right?”

“I think that that created a little bit of mistrust about Illizarov in the early days. They weren't false statements, it was just the way that he looked at things, you know?”

Playing the Winner’s Game in Orthopedics

In business, it’s important to understand what “game” you are playing.

When industries are in their formative stages—think automobiles in the early 20th century, the computer industry in the 1970s, the internet in the 1980s, orthopedics in the 1980s, spine in the 1990s—it is what is colloquially called a “winner’s game.”

In those cases, markets are evolving so fast, that the principal imperative for businesses is to run and gun, also known as blitzkrieg marketing, and gain as much market share as possible, no matter how messy it is. Just clean up as you go.

Later, in the mature stages of an industry—as orthopedics is today—the principal imperative turns 180 degrees from risk taking to risk aversion. Now the strategy is careful planning, no matter how long it takes, and then flawless execution.

The way Richard's head of orthopedics, Ron Pickard, and Lukianov developed the Illizarov was well suited to the "winner's game" phase of orthopedics in the 1980s.

For Lukianov, everything was new. "Richards was my first orthopedic company. My eyes were wide open. I got promoted very, very quickly to run the Illizarov business unit. I knew nothing about how to run a business unit. I don't even know why they promoted me."

"The Richard's culture was it was okay to go out there and swing for the fences. And that was more Ron Pickard than Jack Blair. Ron ran the orthopedic division. The first time I met Ron I thought to myself, you know what? I think I want his job. I like what he does. Richards was interesting then. Ron and the company were all about taking market share. In those days it was a trauma company that was trying to morph itself into a joint company."

"They had the big foray into total knees and total hips, Charnley's hip was just coming out. Then this whole Illizarov thing came about. It was an opportunity for Richards to really be noticed because it got a lot of headlines."

"Remember, back then there was a lot of tension between the U.S. and Russia. We were in a Cold war with Russia back in the eighties. Here we were at

Richards bringing technology out of Russia during the Cold War. That in and of itself was a crazy process."

"I had zero interest in going to Russia. I mean, none. I had no interest in using my Russian language."

Lukianov was from New York originally. His grandparents fled the Russian Revolution in the early part of the 20th century. His paternal grandfather was a white army officer and fought the Bolsheviks all the way across Russia—eventually ending up in Shanghai, China. Lukianov's father was born in Shanghai and lived there until he was 21.

When China's communist party took control of the country after World War II, the Lukianovs fled to the Philippines where they stayed almost two years as displaced persons. Connections with an American Orthodox Russian Archbishop brought the family, via San Francisco, to New York City. Alex's grandfather on his mother's side, was a priest in the Russian Orthodox church at a time when priests were being executed by the Russian authorities. The family was able to escape Russia and settled initially in Poland. Through efforts of the American Red Cross, they also made their way to New York City via Germany.

Alex's parents met in New York at a little storefront, Russian Orthodox Church.

"So, when Rick Treharne, Ron Pickard, and Jack Blair wanted me to go to Russia, I said 'I don't wanna go to Russia.' They insisted. 'Well, you gotta go with us. You can help us.'"

So, the grandson of a white army officer and a Russian Orthodox priest, returned to Russia to negotiate, he hoped, a license deal for the Illizarov external fixator.

"We get to Moscow, and we go to one of the key hotels. We sit down to have dinner. Of course, Jack Blair and the other Richard's engineer want me to translate and explain what's on the menu. I translated the entire menu. The waiter comes over and I give him our order. And then he says 'we don't have that.' I ask about another menu item. 'No, we don't have that either.' Ok, so, of course, we start all over again explaining the menu and order once again to be told they don't have that either."

"So, then I asked, 'What do you have?' He said, 'We have a little beef and some pickles.' This menu was about six pages. And all they have is beef and pickles. Take it or leave it. Of course, Jack and the engineer want to know what has been said. So, I tell the guys 'you're having beef and pickles.'"

"We go from Moscow to Siberia, off the airplane, walk downstairs to the tarmac (no jetway) and the temperature was a fricking 50 below zero. We had no hats on. I mean, you can't even be out there for more than a couple of minutes, right? The Russian guys wore fur hats are laughing at us, and I could hear 'em, 'look at these idiot Americans they have no hats.'"

"Jack ended up buying some kind of really cheap beaver hat, which he thought was a pretty nice fur hat, but it was a really a cheap beaver hat. Every time he wore it, the Russians were saying, 'I can't believe that a president of a big company is wearing that really cheap beaver hat'. But I saw no reason to translate everything I heard."

"After all that, we got nothing done with the Russians. We came back to Memphis and Jack Blair said to me, 'I want you to go over there and negotiate a license.' I'd never negotiated a license in my life. I didn't know the first thing about it."

"I get sent over there, I show up in Moscow, and I go to meet with my counterpart. I ask him, 'where are we gonna meet? Which conference room?' He says, 'Nope, we don't have a conference room, we'll just meet in your hotel room.' Well, they'd put me into a cheap hotel where the rooms have two bunk beds."

“I'm sitting on the bottom of a bunk bed hunched over and so is my counterpart. We're going through our negotiating positions. It was so Bush League, so ridiculous. We're sitting there on these bunk beds negotiating. Pretty soon, it's lunchtime. And the negotiator says ‘Alex, you want to get some lunch?’ I said ‘absolutely’ and we head down to the restaurant.”

“We sit down at the table, and he turns to the waiter and says, ‘Bring us a bottle of vodka.’ The bottles of vodka that they had in Russia had these aluminum pull tops. Once you open a bottle, there’s nothing to reseal it with. So, oh my God, we split a bottle of vodka over lunch. Two of us. I'm absolutely drunk.”

“After lunch, we go back to the bunk beds and are arguing over territories like, we want Chile, but we want Vietnam and I say, ‘you can’t have Vietnam, we fought over Vietnam.’ It was the most ridiculous conversation. We’re going back and forth and I’m thinking ‘this is so pointless.’ And, of course, I’m trying to drink as much coffee as possible.”

“It gets to four o'clock and my counterpart says, ‘Let's go downstairs for a minute.’ And downstairs it’s the same thing all over again. Let's split a bottle of vodka.”

“I've been in Russia for less than 24 hours. I'm have already been drunk twice. Next day, exact same drill, exact lunch, split a bottle of vodka at the end of the day, split a bottle of vodka. I’m thinking ‘I'm gonna die here. I mean, my liver's gonna give out. I'm not gonna make it to day three.’”

“Day three, I'm thinking I have to outsmart this guy. So, I said, I understand that the Georgians make really good wine. I would love to have a glass of wine. He said, ‘Alex, that's a great idea’. Turns to the waiter and says, ‘bring us four bottles of Georgian wine.’”

“I knew that nothing was going to happen that day. My trip basically ended. I came back to Memphis. I returned to Russia two months later, it was completely different. I had been checked out by this guy to see if he liked me or not. I had to give him a lobe of my liver to prove myself. But we actually worked out a deal on educational programs. I found out some ten years later that I had befriended and was negotiating with a Major in the KGB."

Dr. Paley put together a European Traveling Fellowship at the Hospitals of Lecco and Bergamo and other limb lengthening and external fixation centers in Europe, including Kurgan to visit Professor Ilizarov. Richards Medical funded this traveling fellowship.

Lukianov and Richard Treharne, Ph.D., organized a Richards-Ilizarov task force and in June 1986, together with his pregnant wife, Wendy, and 2-year-old son, Ben, Dr. Paley departed for Europe for 6 months which included organizing the inaugural western surgeon trip to the USSR and Kurgan.

Kurgan, where Ilizarov was practicing was a closed city. The fact that Paley had organized a medical conference in Kurgan, allowed Richards and a group of Western surgeons to visit and be trained by the Master himself.

The First Course in Kurgan, Siberia

To this day, Lukianov remembers that first course in Siberia vividly. "At our first course in Siberia, I had prepped all the surgeons to be on their best behavior. I told them that if anything goes wrong for the Americans or Canadians, I swear I will kill you with my own hands. People are gonna hear about what we're doing here because there is still Cold War between the U.S. and Russia."

"And we're bringing surgeons into Siberia of all places to be trained. We show up at the hotel, and all these notable surgeons are heading to their rooms to relax, take showers and so forth after a very long trip to the other side of the world. And there's no hot water."

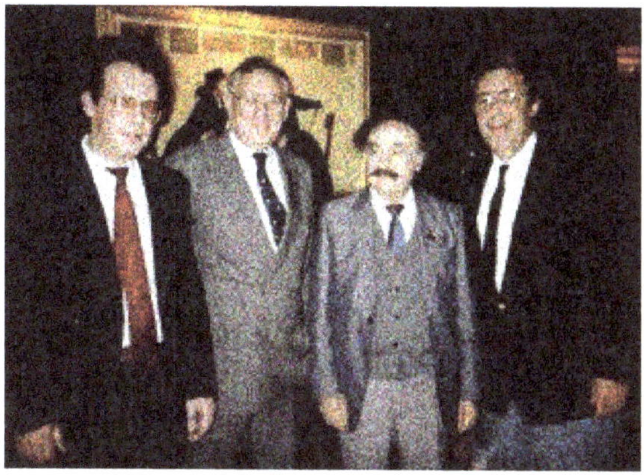

Prof Ilizarov with Victor Frankl and Others

"It was September and there's no hot water in the hotel. I go marching down to the front desk. I tell them that nobody can take a shower. What's going on? And the clerk tells me that the hot water is not turned on until October 15th. I said 'What are you talking about? You mean for the whole city of 360,000 people? Who's in charge? The clerk says, "The Mayor.'"

"So, I went to meet with the mayor. I had just gotten off the airplane the day before and I still had my copy of the *New York Times* with me. I meet with the mayor and introduce myself, 'I'm Alex Lukianov. I'm with this company, Smith & Nephew out of England. And, you know something? I can make you really famous. And the Mayor says, 'What are you talking about?' I said, are you familiar with the *New York Times*? He said, of course, everybody knows the *New York Times*.'"

"I said, I can get you on the front page. He said, 'Are you serious?' I said, absolutely. In the headlines: 'American surgeons come to Siberia, no hot water for showers.' You're gonna be so famous."

By the time I got back to the hotel, they turned on the hot water for the entire city of 360,000 people. It was crazy. After that, every time I asked for something, I got it immediately."

In retrospect, the lessons learned with the Illizarov launch in the U.S.—using educational seminars to teach a new procedure, funding clinical research, and clearly solving an unmet clinical problem—were later repeated with great success with many other new orthopedic and spine products.

For Lukianov himself, he would later follow Ron Pickard to Danek—destined to become the largest supplier of spinal implants, instruments, biologics and robotics ever—and later to take a struggling little spine start up just outside of San Diego named NuVasive and make it the 3rd largest supplier in the world.

CHAPTER NINE: FDA, ASTM AND THE ORTHOPEDIC SURGICAL MANUFACTURER ASSOCIATION

Richards' experience with its modular knee was but one example of the unforeseeable consequences of the phenomenal growth occurring throughout the industry at the time. Yet those consequences were largely due to the innovations described in this book. New designs, new materials, new manufacturing techniques, and new surgical methods usually meant fewer infections and longer-lasting implants for most patients, and some orthopedic implants work better than others.

Conversely, when a procedure did not produce the hoped-for results or when a medical device later failed, complaints were inevitable. And with regard to such failures, it was also inevitable that increased attention would focus on a major difference between the use of orthopedic implant devices and the prescribing of drugs: the latter required extensive testing before being used, the other did not.

Not that orthopedic manufacturers were opposed to industry standards. As far back as 1954, five companies—Richards, DePuy, Zimmer, OEC, and Wright Medical—had formed the Orthopedic Surgical Manufacturers Association (OSMA), with each company represented by its CEO.

Other companies soon joined, and in 1962 OSMA helped create a special committee within the American Society for Testing and Materials to develop standards for materials used in medical and surgical procedures. ASTM had been formed in the late 1890s in response to train accidents caused by rails breaking, and its first action had been to develop standards for steel used in the manufacture of rails.

The new implant standards committee—designated the "F4 Medical and Surgical Materials and Devices Committee" but usually referred to simply as the "F4 Committee"—remains active and includes surgeons, manufacturers, and researchers, but it was never capable of providing a complete solution to increasing concerns about product safety. Only a new regimen, one that prohibited the introduction of insufficiently tested products, could accomplish that.

The FDA Becomes a Power Player in Orthopedics in 1986

Although Congress had intervened in the delivery of health care to the elderly with the enactment of Medicare, it had not provided any mechanism to oversee the quality of medical care that senior citizens—or, for that matter, any patient—actually received, let alone the quality and reliability of orthopedic implants. The widely accepted view was that this was something best left to doctors and their patients, as it always had been.

The only exception to this was the FDA's treatment of the cement used in some hip surgeries: for most purposes, at least initially, the FDA limited use of acrylic cement in hip replacements. Despite Charnley's apparently successful methods using acrylic cement, the FDA classified the product as an "investigational new drug" and restricted its use to licensed surgeons. "This meant that [Charnley's total hip replacement method] could no longer be done without such a license, as the cement was an integral part of the procedure." The Mayo Clinic received the first such license, for experimental use, but that was not until 1969.

Despite the F4 Committee standards, the industry was not subject to any mandatory testing requirements with regard to new devices. Adoption of the standards was an important step, but the committee had no enforcement authority. If a product worked, well and good for all concerned. But if it did not work as intended—which sometimes happened—there was no easy remedy. Medical malpractice litigation was an option, but this was a costly post-injury approach which benefitted few and did little to prevent defective devices coming onto the market. Moreover, problems might not appear immediately—again, Charnley's initial use of PTFE was a classic example. Yet accusations began to mount that "[s]ome medical devices, originally touted as safe and effective, were posing severe health risks to consumers, including death."

What spurred Congress to act, however, was not concern about orthopedic implants. In the early 1970s, the A.H. Robins Company acquired and began marketing the Dalkon Shield, an intrauterine birth control device. It was a popular IUD—some 2.5 million women used it before it was withdrawn from the market in 1974—until complaints began to surface alleging that it was responsible for infections and pelvic inflammatory disease that could lead to infertility. It appeared that the device had undergone only limited testing before being widely marketed as safe and effective. Lawsuits followed, and Robins had to file for bankruptcy, offering to set aside $1.75 billion to compensate women injured by the device. The demand for congressional action proved too great to ignore.

The hands-off approach came to an end in 1976 when Congress enacted the Medical Device Amendments to the Federal Food, Drug, and Cosmetic Act. Among other restrictions, the legislation appeared to mandate prior FDA approval of every new orthopedic implant device before it could be used in any surgery, but the wording of the statute itself was ambiguous in one respect, leaving unanswered an important question that would have to be addressed later. In the meantime, the industry had to contend with a new and complex set of regulations.

To implement the 1976 amendments, FDA regulations categorized all medical devices into three classes, with increasing levels of FDA scrutiny. A Class I device was one that poses a minimum risk to the public (e.g., tongue depressors); these devices would receive minor regulation. A Class II device, one which might result in more harm to patients, would be subject to so-called "special controls." The third category, Class III, would be extensively regulated. A Class III device was defined as one that supports or sustains human life, helps prevent "impairment of human health, or...presents a potential unreasonable risk of illness or injury." This third category included pacemakers, IUDs, and some orthopedic implants.

The increased risk inherent in such devices falling within the third category meant increased scrutiny. New regulations required "Premarket Approval" by the FDA of all new Class III devices "to provide reasonable assurance of its safety and effectiveness." If a device failed to meet FDA standards, it could not be marketed. However, a grandfather provision did exclude from the premarket approval requirement any device on the market before May 28, 1976.

In theory, manufacturers with rigorous testing procedures would have no problem securing approval for safe devices, but actual implementation did not work that way. So many new devices were being developed by the various manufacturers and so many people (both surgeons and patients) were demanding them that it was thought that the FDA might be overwhelmed with applications. And the Premarket Approval procedure (in short form, "PMA") was itself rigorous and time consuming for manufacturers.

An application submitted to the FDA had to include extensive data on clinical testing—testing which required preapproval by the FDA in the first place—and the FDA review of the application routinely took some 1,200 hours. Even when approvals were granted, the FDA would routinely condition its approval on continued annual reports from the manufacturer, reports that required extensive monitoring not only of its own device, but which had to include any information it had regarding similar devices made by competitors.

Orthopedic manufacturers who wanted to avoid the lengthy delays inherent in securing Premarket Approval for new devices—in other words, every orthopedic manufacturer—soon discovered that the 1976 amendments had created a path around the PMA process. In brief, "new" did not always mean *new*. This was because section 510(k) of the 1976 legislation permitted the sale and use of a device if the device was "substantially equivalent" to other products already on the market.

In such instances, no lengthy, formal FDA review of the device was required. In sharp contrast to the hundreds of agency hours expended in the typical PMA process, only 20 agency hours were needed to review each 510(k) submission. This route, called "Premarket Notification," would become the avenue of choice for manufacturers wanting the earliest possible marketing of their "new" implant products.

Not surprisingly, this bypassing of the formal PMA procedure was subject to criticism almost from the start and would eventually lead to further federal legislation. "Substantial equivalence" is an elastic term, and 510(k) products were not subject to the same follow-up notification requirements. Critics would come to brand it a "loophole that allowed untested products onto the market without adequate regulatory oversight." But if it was a loophole, it carried some genuine risks for the manufacturers as well.

Preemption of State Laws

Another feature of the Medical Device Amendments would also have an impact on manufacturers. Prior to the Medical Device Amendments, a patient who believed that he or she had been harmed by a defective orthopedic implant could usually file a lawsuit under state law not only against his or her surgeon, but also against the company which had manufactured the device. State laws typically provided that if it could be shown that a manufacturer knew or should have known that its device posed an undue risk to patients, the company could be held liable for any harm that resulted. In that respect, orthopedic implants were treated the same as other products used by the public.

The Medical Device Amendments changed this, although the extent to which it was changed would not be finally settled until the issues reached the U.S. Supreme Court decades later. Section 360k of the original Act provided that once the FDA promulgates specific requirements as to a device, those FDA requirements "preempt" any state law to the contrary. In other words, if a medical implant device has been specifically approved by the FDA, any state law with regard to such devices was essentially rendered null and void, even those state laws that set higher standards. At least this was true with regard to devices which had gone through the regular Premarket Approval process.

Unanswered—at least not unequivocally answered—was whether the manufacturer of a "510(k)" device, i.e., one allowed onto the market through the Premarket Notification process, could be held liable under state law if the device was shown to be harmful. Did the preemption provision supplant state laws with regard to a device that came onto the market via Premarket Notification? If it did not, a manufacturer who relied on Premarket Notification would still be exposed to liability it would not have incurred had it secured Premarket Approval.

Despite this uncertainty and the risk of liability, manufacturers were quick to utilize the 510(k) process, and this would remain the case, at least until 2006, when the U.S. Supreme Court resolved the issue by holding that state products liability laws were not preempted with regard those 510(k) devices. Statistics for the year just preceding that decision shows just how extensive the practice had become. Of some 3,180 medical implant devices submitted to the FDA that year for all branches of the FDA, only 32 were for formal Premarket Approval. The rest were 510(k) devices submitted through Premarket Notification.

However, this disparity does not necessarily imply that manufacturers were trying to skirt the law, let alone endanger patients. The simple fact was that many "new" devices were so similar to devices already on the market as to be almost copies. With every manufacturer determined to offer as wide a product line as possible in order to be competitive, none of them was going to voluntarily go through what was seen as an unnecessary and time-consuming process.

But even the simpler Premarket Notification process required manufacturers, including Richards, to change how they developed and marketed products. It was no longer enough to avoid infringing upon an existing patent; companies now had to show, through extensive documentation, that a proposed device was truly *substantially equivalent* to one already in use. And at Richards Manufacturing, much of the responsibility for compliance with the new requirements also fell to L.D.

Big Changes at Richards

This may have been partly by default because of increasingly strained relations between Treace and the Rorer management.

For years, Rorer had been content to let Richards operate largely as it had done before the acquisition—why interfere with a company that by all measures was a resounding success?

But that success was predicated on continued growth, and Richards routinely plowed its profits back into new devices, expanded markets, and its own acquisitions. This was all done with Rorer's approval, but the continued expansion by Richards had two interlocked consequences: Rorer was not yet receiving a large return on its investment, and it was no longer satisfied with this arrangement.

There was also the matter of the continuing dispute with Dr. Marmor, which could not have pleased Rorer management regardless of where the true fault lay. It was a distraction and not an inexpensive one.

As for Treace, he began to chafe at what he saw as Rorer's lack of support. There had always been, as L.D. described it, "a kind of guarded relationship" between Treace and Rorer's sometimes contentious CEO, John Eckman, who would not hesitate to point out that even though subsidiaries might still retain their own presidents, but there was only one CEO who was ultimately in charge.

Yet actual intervention by Rorer in operations at Richards was rare, at least at the beginning.

"They actually left us alone for about ten years. John [Eckman] wouldn't fool with it that much. We'd have quarterly meetings and he'd make his comments, but he didn't really get involved. They let that go on for, I guess, close to ten years."

In fact, Eckman had told Treace that they wanted him to continue to run Richards as he always had. But by the mid-1970s the relationship had changed, and Treace's discontent with that change was evident to L.D.:

"By that time, he had just terrible seller's remorse, and he went on about how the biggest mistake he had ever made was selling the company. He was unhappy about that for the rest of his life. I don't think he ever saw the problem as it was."

Treace's unhappiness must have been evident to everyone around him. More than a quarter-century later, his personal secretary, Betty Cole, would remember and also understand Treace's frustrations with Rorer's second-guessing of his decisions:

"Once you've owned a company and been the person who makes the decisions and sets the direction and the culture and the tone of the company, it's very hard to stay on for a long time after a conglomerate like Rorer comes in and takes over the company. You just don't have the same level of 'say' that you had before, and you have to make up your mind that that's the way it's going to be. But for most creative people who are at the top of an organization, it's hard for them to do."

With Treace and the leadership at Rorer often at cross purposes, the spillover began to have an effect on L.D. as well, for he soon had to serve as kind of unofficial liaison between the two companies: "The relationship was getting further and further in trouble. They wouldn't call Harry for anything."

How bad the relationship had deteriorated became apparent to L.D. when Treace spoke to him about hiring a new chief financial officer at Richards. The man Treace had in mind for the job had a strong resume but, in L.D.'s view, was not really suitable for job. He just did not have the practical experience that L.D. thought was needed. Nevertheless, he felt that it should be Treace's decision. Said L.D.: "Well, you're the president. Go ahead. He's not my pick, but if you want him, do it."

Treace's reply came as a shock: "Can't. Rorer won't approve it without your approval."

Thinking "That's a hell of a note," L.D. returned to his office and called Gordon Moyer, Rorer's president. L.D. explained the situation and said he thought that Treace should be able to name his own CFO. Moyer's response was unexpected: Rorer would approve the hire only if L.D. became executive vice president and would oversee the day-to-day operations at Richards.

Fisher had retired, as planned, a year after L.D.'s return to Memphis, but Rorer had not acted immediately to fill the position. Now the position was

L.D.'s without even having to ask. He accepted, but it turned out to be a temporary arrangement.

The management at Rorer must have been pleased with L.D.'s accomplishments as executive vice president because only a year after his promotion the same management decided to impose a drastic change in the leadership at Richards. Given the tortuous relationship between Rorer and Treace, it is unlikely that L.D. was totally surprised when Moyer, still Rorer's president, called to tell him of their plan. He came right to the point:

"Harry will be 62 years old. We would like to create a new position of chairman of Richards and put him as chairman, but you take over as president with full operating responsibility and authority."

As always when faced with an important decision, L.D. went home to discuss it with Betty. They went for a long walk and considered the options. Both agreed that he could not turn down the offer, but L.D. told her that his chances of staying with Richards until retirement had decreased by 75%. There were just too many unresolved issues, including a libel suit judgment against Richards (by Marmor) then on appeal. Although Richards Manufacturing was doing well by every measure, other things were up in the air, including the company's future relationship with Rorer.

In fact, L.D. had few doubts as to where that was heading. Even as L.D. was being asked to head Richards, Rorer was hiring managers at the corporate level to review and approve decisions that had once been the province of its subsidiaries. Rorer had a new vice president of personnel who would now oversee decisions by local personnel managers, and there was a new corporate vice president in charge of Rorer's Medical Division. Rorer's "tentacles," as L.D. would later label them, were bound to increase.

On January 1, 1979, the man who had joined Richards Manufacturing as a shipping clerk some nineteen years earlier—and had even had to ask what an implant was—became the company's third president.

Treace Is Replaced, L.D. Beard Becomes President

It is unknown whether Treace was surprised by Rorer's decision, but it must have been very difficult for him to leave the company he had built into a worldwide competitor in the orthopedic implant industry. When he had sold Richards in 1968 he could not have envisioned that things could ever come to such a pass.

For nearly twenty-three years—fifteen as company president—Treace had been the person, the force really, primarily responsible for new product designs at Richards. No one was more mindful of this than L.D., and one of his first decisions was to make sure that the company's development of new products did not suffer.

Even if Treace was no longer active within the company, he had left behind two important legacies—L.D., whose talents he had spotted early, and Treace's son Jim, who had inherited many of his father's skills in product design and development. L.D. named him executive vice president and placed him in charge of new products.

Under L.D.'s leadership, Richards would continue to grow and add significant new devices to its product line. Perhaps ironically, the patent application for one of these had been filed by Harry Treace just before he was removed as president: this was Richards' Total Ossicular Replacement Prosthesis (TORP). Like one the first major devices that Treace had developed at Richards, it was designed to remedy hearing loss. That first one, co-developed with Dr. Shea, had been a replacement for a tiny bone called a stapes; the new prosthesis was designed to replace other adjacent tiny bones that had degenerated, and it incorporated a movable joint to make the surgical procedure easier.

A second successful device was called the Richards Fixation Staple. Bone staples had been in use for decades, but the Richards device was a new approach to a recurrent problem: "holding the staples in the proper location as they are driven into and/or removed from bone structure." The Richards invention—credited to Calvin Griggs in the patent application—was a significant advance, consisting of a grooved staple and an improved staple holder.

Again, the sales numbers chronicled the company's growth. The total net sales for 1991 reached $69 million, an increase of some 50% over the 1978 figure. But this did not ease the troubled relationship with Rorer, which was playing out much as L.D. had expected.

He did not like being second-guessed any better than Treace had, especially by corporate suits who would visit Richards but who knew far less about the orthopedic industry than he did.

Especially galling was an assertion by one such visitor that none of the subsidiaries had management in place that was capable of leading them into the 1980s.

After two years of this sort of thing, the usually mild-mannered L.D. decided to share his thoughts about Rorer's intrusions into what had always been local decision making. A quarterly meeting at Rorer was just about to close when L.D. said that he had something to add:

"I have been called, criticized, spent 40% of my time on the phone with [the vice president in charge of surgical product and the vice president of personnel] criticizing everything. I've done pretty well with people in the past, and so I've just made up my mind anytime that you call and want to talk about people I'm going to hang up the phone. I'm not going to talk to you about it. Either I'm running it, or I'm not."

Moyer was taken aback but no resolution was reached and probably could not have been reached. This was because underlying the surface elements was a fundamental difference in goals: although Richards was paying Rorer large management fees, Rorer wanted more. That it owned an extraordinarily valuable subsidiary did not appear to count all that much.

In August, things came to a head again when L.D. traveled to Rorer's main offices seeking a temporary loan for some construction projects. This was not unusual, and Richards would repay the loan at the end of the year. But this time Rorer refused.

To L.D., this attitude was inexplicable because Richards was then working on a new total hip prosthesis using a new material, which was requiring some major outlays. However, now that he had been rebuffed by Rorer, L.D. had no choice but to cancel the project in order to conserve cash. He informed Rorer's vice president in charge of surgical products of his plans but was surprised at a subsequent meeting when Eckman, Rorer's CEO, accosted him about his decision, accusing L.D. of trying to embarrass him.

This was too much. L.D. replied that the project had become a cash drain and that it was his job to cut out cash drains. The tone of the conversation, if that is the right term, did not improve.

When Eckman then told L.D. that he should have called him first, L.D. pointed out that under the new management structure he did not report directly to Eckman, but to a corporate vice president.

Eckman, who did not like challenges to his authority, retorted that L.D. should have at least called that person.

Said L.D., "Well, in fact I did."

"When," asked Eckman angrily, "Yesterday?"

L.D. must have enjoyed his own rejoinder: "The day I did it. Before I made the decision."

Only then did the corporate vice president in question—who had sat by silently while L.D. was being berated by Eckman—speak up and confirm that L.D. had indeed called him as L.D. had stated.

But being right can have consequences, as L.D. surely was aware: "Once these things had transpired, I knew that my days were numbered."

When he later told Betty about the confrontation, her attitude was "Why not just quit and go somewhere else?"

Not yet, thought L.D.

It was not long before the inevitable happened. At another meeting at Rorer, it was announced that Treace's three-year term as board chairman would end the following year and that L.D. would be named to replace him. The impolite term is "kicked upstairs," but L.D. was not unhappy. He now had other plans.

CHAPTER TEN: SPINE SURGERY BECOMES A SPECIALTY

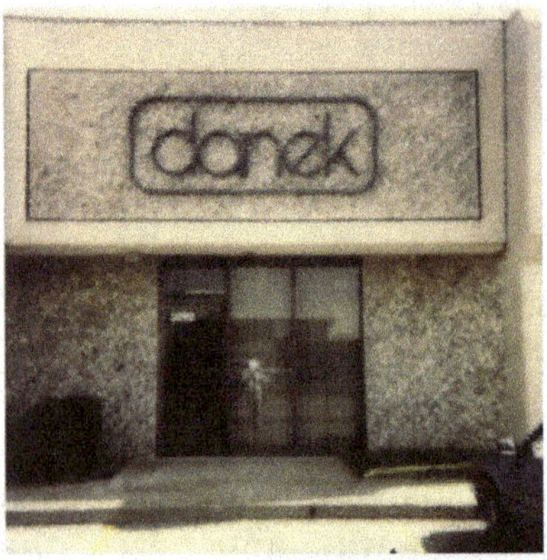

Danek Medical's first location, in a strip mall near Richards.

Alan Olsen and Dr. Eduardo Luque, circa 1988

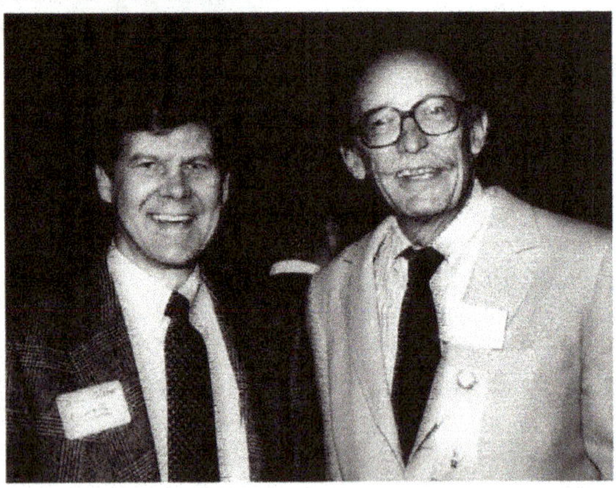

In 1986 Rorer sold Richards Manufacturing to Parker Montgomery and CooperVision for $350 million. A few years later, London based Smith & Nephew bought the firm and operates the facility on Brooks Road to this day.

All of those managerial changes took a toll on the Richards' management team. At one point, one of the owners asked for each senior manager's curriculum vitae, you know, to judge the capabilities of the people they had working for them.

Soon after Harry Treace left, his sons followed.

In the end, L.D. Beard took his wife's advice to "go somewhere else," but it was not in his nature to act impulsively. He wanted to make sure it was the right "somewhere else." He could not have known where his choice would lead.

What L.D. had learned during the year he was chairman of Richards' board was that he was not well suited to the position: "I was chairman, which was sort of, I guess, historian and chief ribbon cutter. That's about what it amounted to. A big office and a good title." But titles had never meant much to L.D.

L.D. wanted to go in a new direction, one that he had thought about more than once during his years at Richards. He had been responsible for a number of acquisitions for his employer, typically involving stock worth several millions of dollars, and he had learned about the history and growth of those smaller companies, their management, and their strengths and weaknesses.

"I looked at the companies and what they'd done, and I thought, I believe I could do that."

And it was not over-confidence on his part. He not only knew the business inside out—he had done it all, from shipping clerk to CEO—he had spent a lot of time thinking about what he knew.

Even before he had anything specific in mind, in 1983 he told Gordon Moyer, Rorer's president, that he might be leaving before his contract ended the following year. Moyer's main concern was the possibility of competition, and L.D. acknowledged that it could happen, adding that this was the business that he knew and that there was no non-compete provision in his contract. So, when the right opportunity presented itself, events moved quickly.

The Beginning of Modern Spine Surgery

Pittsburgh, Youngstown, Akron, Cleveland, and Detroit, the cities of America's great industrial heartland, were, in 1978, shedding plants and employees like so much excess baggage in a desperate fight for economic survival. Newspaper headlines captured the angst of the moment with the "Pain Index"—which was the rate of inflation added to the rate of unemployment.

The year started in Cleveland with the "blizzard of the century" which blew through these rust belt cities (82 mph wind gusts) leaving 20 foot snow drifts, 60-below wind chills and 51 people dead in and around Cleveland.

The year ended with the city defaulting on $15 million in debt—the first major U.S. city to do so. Cleveland's police refused to patrol crime hot spots—despite Mayor Dennis Kucinich's order to do so. Too risky, they said.

And yet, in one of the most dangerous sections of Cleveland, at a hospital named "Charity", three orthopedic surgeons were planning something that would eventually form the basis and structure of modern spine surgery.

Karl Alfred, Arthur Steffee, and Dennis Stuart

Karl Alfred was head of the Orthopedics Department at St. Vincent's Charity Hospital in one of the more economically distressed and crime ridden sections of Cleveland. Art Steffee was his partner and Dennis Stuart was a resident.

Across town, at the tonier Cleveland Clinic—A. Seth Greenwald, D.Phil.(Oxon), had established one of the early orthopedic laboratory and surgeon education programs in the United States which, with the advent of the Charnley hip and the associated hip arthroplasty procedure, was an increasing popular program among aspiring orthopedic surgeons.

The orthopedics program, at the Cleveland Clinic Foundation (aka: The Clinic), however, was missing one critical element—trauma training.

One of the busiest emergency rooms in the region was at St. Vincent's Charity Hospital. As Art Steffee himself would later say about Charity Hospital's neighborhood, "We have bullets flying around here like mosquitos."

A perfect match evolved. Cleveland Clinic's orthopedic residents rotated through Charity for trauma training.

Greenwald organized a monthly lecture series, inviting surgeons from all over the United States and Europe, the who's who of orthopedics at the time, to the Cleveland Clinic, while always including Karl Alfred's group from Charity—which, as time passed, proved to be an irritant to The Clinic.

As Greenwald's relationship with The Clinic grew strained, Greenwald began thinking about starting his own laboratory and education institute. He shared his ideas with the Charity group and in 1980, Alfred, Steffee, and Stuart made a proposal to support Greenwald's dream by guaranteeing his salary and rounding up funding beyond his existing NIH, DoD and corporate grants for equipment, an animal facility, a cadaver lab, a full biomechanics and fabrication facility, a surgical suite and more.

Greenwald agreed and, in the spring of 1981, with much fanfare, the Cleveland Research Institute (CRI) was born.

Testing, Training and Fabrication

CRI was an independent corporation housed in newly remodeled research building adjacent to St. Vincent's Charity Hospital. Seth Greenwald was Director. Charity's president, David D'Eramo said at the time, that CRI would "enhance Cleveland's already superlative medical reputation" by becoming a focal point for ideas and a forum to attract scientists from "near and far." Good news at a time when Cleveland was better known for unemployment, crime and a river that caught fire.

But one man, above all, would use CRI as the launching pad for the first modern spinal implant company, AcroMed, and, using Greenwald's structure, equipment, and personnel to create the R&D and intellectual property foundation for future spine surgery implants, procedures, and instruments.

Arthur Steffee.

Along with his equipment, all of the engineering graduate students and staff from his lab at the Cleveland Clinic followed Greenwald to CRI. James Moran, who would complete his Ph.D. while working at CRI, headed up the engineering staff. Sue Martin administered CRI's education courses for residents and visiting surgeons. Twenty, thirty or more physicians attended each of the classes. Among the students was a young Gary Michelson, a surgeon who would become one of the most prolific and controversial spinal implant inventors ever.

CRI engineers Andy Cepulo, Jack Geiger, Diane Peterson, Joe Skraba, and Terry Stahurski as well as Eileen Morgan (who was also in charge of the animal lab and assisted in surgery and cadaver labs) joined

Greenwald and were integral to the innovative products flowing out of CRI. Jim Berry, who had a master's in biology, carried out histology and tissue culture work, collaborating on foundational research on the implant-bone interface.

And then there was Frank Janson.

Greenwald literally found him in the Cleveland Clinic's maintenance department, in the hospital's basement. Greenwald recalls, "He was quite an adept guy. I liked him a lot. He was a crack machinist. And we produced a lot of equipment together. You didn't need to give Frank blueprints. In fact, if you gave him blueprints, it got in the way. He had a lot of creative ideas. He developed a lot of the equipment we had in the lab."

Stahurski recalls, "Frank Janson was brilliant, he could make anything, anything you wanted, and improve it too."

Indeed, Frank Janson may well be the unsung hero of the first widely commercialized spinal implant: The Steffee Plate. But we are getting ahead of the story.

Spinning Ideas and Concepts

It was the early days of biomedical engineering and there was really not the specialization that exists today...interface experts, biomaterial experts. CRI's staff each had training in specific areas, but because the lab was dependent on soft money, in order to pay the bills, CRI's staff took on a wide variety of projects.

As Terry Stahurski recalls; "There was a lot of innovation at CRI. Everyone had 3 or 4 projects going on at any one time. Things that are taken for granted now, were unknown then. The patents and intellectual property were wide open. We were paid next to nothing and one of CRI's main tenets was to keep one particular surgeon happy, Art Steffee."

Among the implants, instruments and testing equipment that initiated at The Clinic's Biomechanics Laboratory and further developed at CRI were:

- A suction lavage machine
- A shoulder resurfacing system including implants and instrumentation.
- Testing fixtures and test methods for bovine tendon and ligament xenografts
- Spinal vertebral plates
- A pneumatically powered bone grinder
- A multi-axial wrist replacement
- Novel acrylic bone cement additives as well as antibiotics for use with artificial joints
- Porous surfaces to promote bone growth.
- Custom tool modifications for Occupational Therapy
- New testing equipment, fixtures, and testing methods for orthopedic tissue
- Ongoing surgical instrument sharpening and repair for the entire hospital

But, perhaps the most enduring aspect of CRI was its commitment to education and training. "We had the residents come through the lab as part of their rotation. They would come up with projects.", remembers Jim Moran. "The younger ones would come in with fresh eyes and they would say 'why the heck are you doing that?' and 'could we do this better?' or 'this is a problem that I saw in surgery today. Is there something we can do about it?'"

At its peak, between administration, orthopedics, cardiovascular and a clinical research coordinating office, CRI had about 35 or 40 employees.

Fabricating an Implant for Steffee *DURING* Surgery

As Stahurski recalls, "Steffee was always bringing ideas to CRI. He'd say 'I need a patellar tendon' or whatever. But you had to watch him because if you had a prototype, he might think it was good enough for implantation."

One story in particular illustrates CRI's dynamic, creative, get-it-done culture.

It was Friday afternoon, about 1pm. Dr. Steffee had a patient on the table, sedated and ready to receive an entire, titanium femur replacement. The implant had been fabricated by an outside firm, Techmedica.

As Steffee tried to lay the implant into the gap he'd created by removing the patient's femur, he found it wouldn't fit. Apparently, when Steffee gave the company the dimensions for the replacement part, he'd applied a magnification factor. The company then also applied that same magnification factor—resulting in a too-long implant.

With an open, sedated patient lying on the table, Steffee called Techmedica. What they could do, they said, was fabricate a replacement part, take it to the airport and put it on a plane.

Steffee hung up the phone and ran to CRI.

Frank Janson, Jim Moran, and Jack Geiger broke the task into components and started working in parallel. The center of the implant was hollow, so they cut a section out from the middle. They fabricated a dowel which fit into the hollow core, pinned it across, welded it, bead blasted it and passivated what was now a precisely fitted implant. In less than two hours, start to finish, Janson and his team got the replacement implant up to the operating room.

The following Monday, Dr. Steffee wheeled his femur replacement patient down to the lab to introduce the team to the patient and vice versa.

The First Implanted Artificial Human Vertebrae

In 1984, a 54-year old woman on her way back to Cleveland from a 500-mile driving trip out west, felt a pulling, then an excruciating pain in her back. The cause, she would soon learn, was a spinal tumor which, for her survival, needed to be removed and with it, one of her vertebrae.

She was referred to St. Vincent's and Dr. Steffee, who was now head of the hospital's Orthopedics Department.

After reviewing her case, Steffee decided that he and the CRI team could, using the patient's X-rays to calculate its dimensions, fabricate a prosthetic vertebra which would maintain her spine's stability and lordotic structure. If he was right, he would be inventing the world's first vertebral prosthesis.

On October 25, 1985, in a 5-hour operation, which had to be delayed one week while the CRI engineers finished making the implant, Steffee removed the cancerous bone and replaced it with a titanium spacer, two Steffee plates and multiple pedicle screws.

Frank Janson made the implant with design input from Jim Moran and Jack Geiger. Originally Steffee wanted polyethylene plugs in the construct into which he'd insert bone screws. Jim Moran suggested that they, instead, put polyethylene cylinders and that they pre-drill the cylinders to accept the pedicle screw. That way, Steffee could put the screws in and rotate the cylinder within the vertebral body which would let him line the screws up with the two Steffee plates (five or six slots).

Helen Murphy and the artificial vertebrae

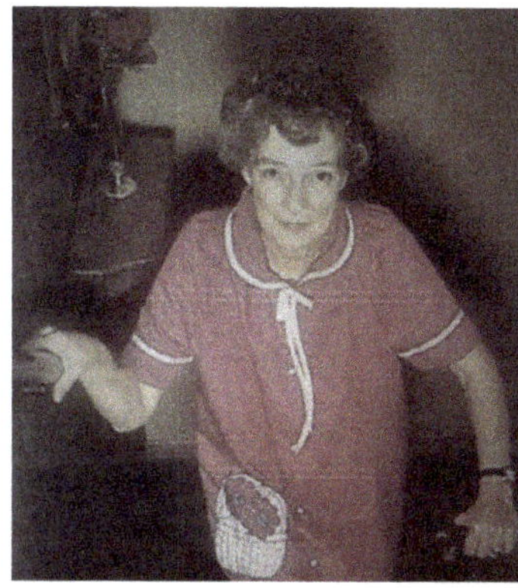

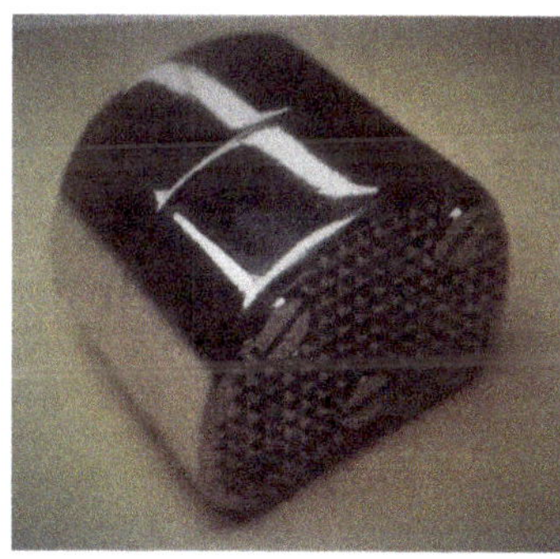

Source: St. Vincent's Charity Hospital and Health Center

The operation was so successful that St. Vincent's issued a press announcement about this important surgical "first" and asked the patient, Helen Murphy, to describe to the media how she was feeling. She told the reporters, "I was hopeful and confident in the surgery; it was my only chance. It's hard to believe that the artificial vertebra is really there because I don't feel it. I was walking a week after surgery and was home in 10 days. It was worth it all just to be able to walk again."

Helen's husband, Richard Murphy, praised Dr. Steffee saying, "He gave Helen back her life."

The Steffee Plate

In 1981, Art Steffee had an idea for a variable screw placement plate and screw system which gave surgeons a comparatively easy way to place bone screws precisely into the center of each pedicle while also providing a way to angulate each screw. The Steffee Plate made configuration of the construct more dependent on the patient's own spinal anatomy than on the limitations of the plates themselves.

The Steffee Plate would become the first mass commercialized spinal implant and the basis for the first purely spinal implant company—AcroMed.

In that post-World War II era, starting with Harrington's posterior rods, then continuing with Luque's modifications to the rod and his segmental sublaminal wiring and evolving further with Roy-Camille's posterior spine plates with transpedicular bone screws, surgery to correct deformity and instability was taking hold, slowly. Patient outcomes, while still hampered by too much pseudoarthrosis, long periods of immobilization and often inadequate decompression, were significantly better than they were pre-World War II.

The Steffee Plate was the game changer which opened up spine surgery as a viable specialty unto itself.

Before the Steffee Plate, surgeons could only insert screws through holes in metal plates. Steffee's variable screw placement (VSP) system reversed that order. Now, surgeons put the screws in first—at whatever angulation they wanted—then laid the plates over the screws where they'd put a nut over the screw head. Also, instead of holes, the VSP plate had slots which allowed for variability based on the patient's anatomy. The slots, in turn, had nests which captured and held the nut to the screw.

The VSP screws also had both a cancellous thread section and a machine threaded section for securing the nut. Before this, bone screws were either threaded for cortical (harder) bone or cancellous (softer) bone.

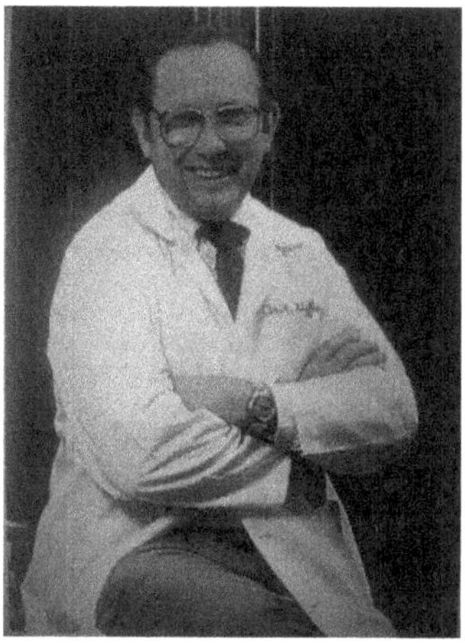

Art Steffee M.D. circa 1990

CRI's engineering team took Art's vision and added a number of key features. It was, according to those who were there at the time, a collaborative effort. Frank Janson made the first prototypes. Jim Moran led the engineering effort. Joe Skraba did the drawings. And the final VSP system was, in fact, the work product of Steffee, the CRI engineers, and Greenwald together.

One day Steffee literally took the plates, the VSP screws and instrumentation from CRI and in collaboration with Ed Wagner, a venture capitalist and local businessman, started a company named AcroMed. Almost simultaneously, he filed for a patent (December 16, 1983) and roughly three weeks later, assigned it to AcroMed.

Patent number 4611581 was granted by the U.S. Patent and Trade Office (PTO) on September 16, 1986, naming Steffee as sole inventor. Three years later, March 29, 1989, to be exact, AcroMed licensed the Steffee plate to a Memphis-based start-up company named Danek Medical.

Frank Janson, who was not listed on the patent believed that he was, in fact, responsible for Claim 8 of Steffee's patent (which described a "surface means for engaging said nut [as described in Claim 7] against sidewise movement relative to said plate as said nut rotated to said force transmitting member [pedicle screw]."

Janson then assigned his claimed ownership of patent 4611581 to Danek Medical in 1995. Later that year, Danek filed a petition with the PTO challenging Steffee's claim that he was sole inventor.

Danek and Janson lost that challenge. On April 12, 1995, the PTO affirmed that Steffee was the sole inventor of the Steffee Plate, patent #4611581.

The End of CRI

Greenwald challenged the unfolding events and was terminated and locked out of CRI in December 1983. All of his grant-purchased equipment which was used to qualify the VSP plates and screws, as well as the library and files brought to CRI at its founding were returned to Greenwald three years later, who was now at Mt. Sinai Medical Center in Cleveland. Art Steffee continued his practice at St. Vincent's while also launching AcroMed.

In retrospect, the beginning of AcroMed was the ending of CRI. A lot of the testing that CRI would otherwise have done for Steffee began going to other places. CRI's finances, which were heavily dependent on government funding, deteriorated. Several CRI engineers left to join Steffee at AcroMed.

One person who did not follow Steffee was Jim Moran, who was then appointed Director of Orthopedic Research at CRI. Today, as he looks back, he notes, "The process worked, we gave life to a very successful company. You would have thought since we helped create the pie, made it grow, we would have gotten a slice. But we didn't. Maybe we could have been a little bit smarter. But the conflicting interests of CRI, St. Vincent's, AcroMed and Dr. Steffee tied our hands. And the lack of support showed exactly how much we were valued."

Having said that, Moran remembers his time working with Steffee fondly. "Art Steffee was interesting. Always had a lot of good ideas. If he was doing something and saw that it wasn't working right, he was the type of person who would recognize that it needed to be improved. Dr. Steffee was a pioneer. You can tell the pioneers because they got the arrows in their back."

Eventually it become too much of a struggle to keep CRI going and it closed quietly a few years later. AcroMed was purchased by DePuy, Inc. in 1998 for $325 million.

R. Lew Bennett, a Richards' employee, kicked off the next great event in the start of modern spine surgery when he told L.D. Beard about a conversation he had had with Dr. George F. Rapp, an Indianapolis orthopedic surgeon.

The Mid-America Orthopaedic Association was in the process of forming—both men would be among its co-founders—and it was at an organizational meeting that they spoke. Dr. Rapp had asked Bennett if he knew of anyone who was available that had the experience to run an orthopedic company. He and some other investors were interested in forming one. Bennett said that he indeed did know just the man, one that ordinarily would not be available, but who might be available now.

L.D. was available, and he soon became interested.

The orthopedic company Rapp was referring to was a small manufacturer that had been founded in the 1950s in Warsaw, Indiana, by Miles Igo and, at the time, fabricated pins, wires, screws, intermedullary nails and generic soft goods.

Besides Dr. Rapp and Miles Igo, the other investor was Charles Davis, a real estate developer in Indianapolis. Together, the three men had formed a new company, Biotechnology, Inc., of which Warsaw Orthopedic would be its main subsidiary. Davis, the largest stockholder, was chairman and CEO. What they needed was someone to oversee operations.

Even though it would mean a 60% pay cut for L.D., he and the investors soon reached an agreement for him to become president and chief operating officer, and in August 1993 L.D. resigned as chairman of Richards. Before the year was out, Beard would become the company CEO. It would be a challenge, as L.D. would later recall:

"The company was doing, I think, somewhere between two and three million dollars a year in sales volume and barely breaking even. We had a little over a million dollars borrowed. That was at the time of the high interest rates. About 18.5% was what I think we were paying, but we were generating enough money to keep the note current. But it was a big problem trying to get it off the ground and get it started and get a sales force. We started building a sales force and start building a product line."

At the time, products made by Biotechnology in Warsaw consisted of soft goods (slings, etc.) and OEM subcontract work for larger companies. "OEM" stands for Original Equipment Manufacturer, the name given to a company which manufactures products to be later sold by another company.

Although the plant would be in Warsaw, the main office was in Memphis, as neither L.D. nor Betty wanted to move again. They had done that once, to Mississippi, and this time Betty was especially concerned about the impact that moving would have on their children, who were still in school. She also had grown up in a small town and knew from experience that school choices were limited in a small town. She did not want their children to have to go through another adjustment.

"We had changed from Memphis to Mississippi, and back to Memphis again. I really did not really want to interrupt that again. And truly, I, myself, did not want to move from the South. It was just not a situation I felt I'd be happy in."

So, the Beards remained in Memphis, and Biotechnology maintained its sales office in Warsaw, Indiana.

Of course, this meant a lot of travel on L.D.'s part: "I would be in Indiana at least a week a month, and some months I would go up, come back home, and go back up again."

Usually, he would drive to Warsaw, a twelve-hour trip, just to save on travel costs. At this juncture, cash flow was a greater issue than his time, so he would use the time to dictate memos and notes which he would later play back. It helped him in setting priorities, a necessity now that he was no longer on a virtually unlimited budget as had been the case at Richards. But L.D. was not discouraged even as he reflected on the task before him.

"It's tough starting from scratch, but it will tell me whether or not that my going from the shipping department to the presidency at Richards was a fluke or not. [And] for a while I thought it was, too, as we kept having these challenges."

Then came the fire.

The Fire

Just nine months after L.D. joined Biotechnology, Igo called him with some bad news: there had been a fire at the plant. L.D. was in Memphis at the time and asked about the level of damage. It was "pretty bad," said Igo. L.D. said he would leave immediately. A quarter century later L.D. would still remember what Igo said next:

"Bring whatever inventory you have down there up with you because we don't have anything."

Betty was at work at Hutchinson School that morning when he called to tell her about the fire, and she was likewise alarmed: "Although he didn't say how bad it was, I could tell by the sound of his voice how bad it was. In fact, he said very little other than that everything had burned, and he was headed to Warsaw."

The fire had indeed been bad. One entire section of one building and the entire production facilities for manufacturing soft goods had gone up in flames. The company's entire inventory. The machine shop, which was in another building, had not caught fire, although there was some smoke damage. The cause of the fire was never determined.

Compounding the extent of the disaster was the fact that although the buildings' contents were insured, the individual buildings were not. Nor did the company have business interruption insurance.

Both Betty and L.D. later agreed that her employment at Hutchinson School was fortuitous—they had a son in college—and Betty in particular was pleased: "It wasn't something that I had to do at the time, but when that happened, I was glad I had a job. It sort of paid the tuition, at least."

Hard Choices

Igo and Dr. Rapp wanted to rebuild, but Davis wanted to shut down the operation and use the proceeds from the contents insurance to pay off bank loans. L.D. was somewhere in the middle but would later say that Davis was probably right from a business standpoint, but at the time there simply was no agreement. Which worried the bankers.

L.D. would not forget the uncertainty and the risks:

"We couldn't really agree, and the bankers were getting very anxious, as you can well imagine they might be. And so I came up with the idea that each of us would put in, on an as-needed and when-needed basis, each of the three of us left—we were capable of doing it—$75,000 apiece until we got the insurance settlement on an as-needed and when-needed basis."

Davis was not involved in negotiations with the bank and would ultimately leave the company. This left Igo, Dr. Rapp, and L.D. And it was L.D. who presented the plan to the bank.

No, the bankers said, "as needed and when needed" would not satisfy them. They wanted the $225,000 in the bank, up front. The two sides were at an impasse, so at one meeting L.D. decided to simply matters:

"I told them we weren't going to do that. And they said, 'Well, do you have a choice?' And I put on an act. I asked Miles, 'Do you have a key to the place?' And he said yes, and I laid them on the table. I got up and I said, "Now you fellows are going to be in the orthopedic business and I'm going to go back to Memphis and get a real job. And I hope you enjoy the orthopedic business. It's a lot of fun."

He was literally walking toward the door when the bankers asked him to wait a minute:

"They agreed to whatever we were going to do. Backed down completely and agreed to whatever we were going to do. They'd just hold off until we got everything settled, and so we did. We didn't have any money left, and we didn't have any production facilities, but we were able to pay off the outstanding loan and start all over again. And they gave us a good line of credit going back out again."

The frequency of L.D.'s visits to Warsaw did not increase, but he did start using air travel. He would fly into Indianapolis, then drive a rental car 125 miles to Warsaw. He often had to work late at the plant, and he would then have to rush to make his flight. And driving on Indiana's two-late state roads could be both frustrating and revealing:

"I'd be rushing down on those, and I'd be coming through those little towns, and there'd be a farmer in a pickup truck that would have me blocked. I'd be impatient and I'd drive by him, and I'd look, and I'd say he's not any older than I am. I ought to be doing that. I ought to be going into town for dinner instead of trying to rush and catch a plane."

L.D.'s work habits remained unchanged since his days at Richards, according to Betty:

"His main time to think was late at night where he worked with an adding machine and a pencil. He sat and did the numbers and thought. That was when he worked it out."

This was typical of L.D.'s work philosophy: "to take things as they are and look at them realistically. Look at them realistically and say, okay, what can we do? What are our choices. And then make the best one you can."

Danek

In 1980, Alan Olson, the former Richard's group product director for total joints as well as soft goods and the veterinary product line, founded Danek in 1980 as an orthopedic soft goods company.

Alan Olsen was born in Minnesota and grew up Richfield, a 1st tier, mostly Scandinavian suburb of Minneapolis. From a young age, he'd wanted to be a doctor. He took pre-med courses during his stint as a U.S. Navy corpsman and managed to wrangle a part-time job at Fairview Hospital in Minneapolis, Minnesota. By sheer coincidence, he was assigned to work with Dr. John Moe, one of the most consequential surgeons, instructors and leaders in spine surgery and founder and past president of the Scoliosis Research Society (SRS).

That experience gave Olsen a solid grounding in the still nascent practice of spine surgery.

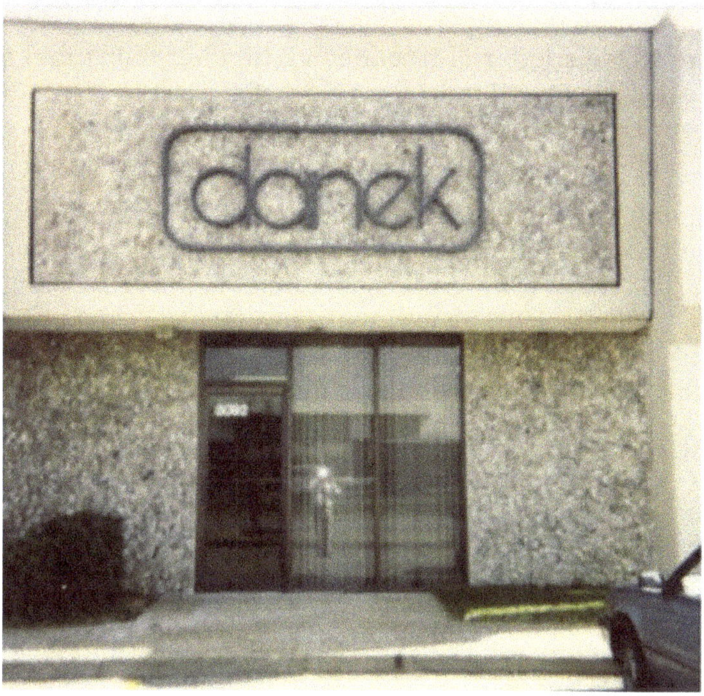

Danek Medical's first location, in a strip mall near Richards

Olsen applied to medical school, supported by Dr. Moe, who wrote a letter of recommendation but didn't make the cut. Disappointed, Olsen opted for work that would keep him in hospitals and working with surgeons—selling medical devices for Richards Manufacturing.

Another seminal moment in Olsen's life and, therefore, the creation of Danek, was when Olsen met with two Galveston, Texas surgeons, Ben Allen and Ron Ferguson, in 1979 about an improvement to the Luque Rod for scoliosis surgery. The Luque rod and sublaminar wiring technique was an alternative to the Harrington Rod and was being marketing by Zimmer.

As Olsen remembers; "Spine was not that big of a thing. But, after listening to Ben Allen and Ron Ferguson, I got really excited. I worked about six months on a presentation to Harry Treace and the Richards' Executive Committee about the Luque rod system improvements. Harry sat back in his chair and said, 'Alan, I know you worked really hard in this project. But if it goes in the brain or spine, we don't do it.'"

Alan and Richards parted ways the day before Thanksgiving, 1979.

"I told my wife, 'Okay, I'm fired'. And she said, 'What?' I said, "Yeah, fired." "Well, what are you going to do?" "I think I'm gonna start a company."

Danek was officially founded by Alan Olsen in January 1980—to, amazingly, make super cheap, mail order arm slings and other orthopaedic soft goods.

How did that work out? Not so well.

"I invested the last $2,000 I had on a direct mail piece that went out on promoting an arm sling that was our first product. After the campaign was out, I went by the mailbox. There's no mail. No return cards. I waited and waited. And finally, after a couple of weeks, I said, "Oh, this isn't working". I got one $75 order out of that whole campaign."

So, Alan tells his wife, "I gotta sell the Corvette. We got to cut some expenses."

He hit the road, knocking on hospital doors. At Memphis Children's Hospital, one of the nurses asked Olsen if he could make restraints to safely protect kids after surgery. He could and did. That patented wrist restraint effectively launched and sustained Danek those first few years.

L.D. Beard and Alan had been talking about going into business together for some time. Shortly after L.D. Beard was able to get Biotechnology back up and running, albeit on a limited basis, he broached the idea of tucking Danek into Biotechnology and having Alan run sales and marketing. "I was thrilled to be doing that," recalls Olsen, "because I couldn't afford to buy old machines to manufacture metal implants, but I could afford to buy sewing machines to make soft goods."

Biotechnology bought Danek Medical in February 1985.

The Luque Screw

In the latter part of 1985, Olsen was contacted by one of Biotechnology's East Coast distributors, John Agricola. A customer, Dr. Ed Simmons, was having issues with the early Zielke rod and screw spinal implants.

Dr. Simmons (1926–1990) was chief of orthopedic surgery at Buffalo General Hospital, future President of the Scoliosis Research Society, Cervical Spine Research Society and Professor of Orthopedic Surgery, University of Toronto and SUNY at Buffalo.

Alan, who had trained with another founder of the Scoliosis Research Society, Dr. John Moe, flew to New York to meet Dr. Simmons.

In a hot, cramped room in Buffalo General Hospital, Alan sat down with Dr. Simmons and about a half dozen of his spine fellows. Simmons, as Olsen remembers, was throwing up X-rays saying, here's what's happening in my surgical spine cases: "on this one, the screws are breaking", "on this one, the rod is breaking".

So, Alan asked him, "Dr. Simmons, how many of these things do you use and how much do they cost?" Simmons told him. So, Olsen did a simple calculation, and he about fell off the chair. Dr. Simmon's usage would totally blow away Biotechnology's annual sales numbers with just Buffalo General's spinal implant purchases.

From Buffalo, New York, Alan flew to Indianapolis for a Biotechnology Board Meeting with Dr. George Rapp and L.D. Beard. On the plane ride back, Olsen sketched out the rough design of an implant that *might* solve Ed Simmon's spine implant problems. It was a bone screw that clamped onto a rod at various angles.

As Alan was describing his meeting with Dr. Ed Simmons and showing them his sketches, George Rapp was amazed "Holy cow. You met with Ed, you know, we almost became partners. Alan," said Dr. Rapp, "if you want to get into spine, you need to go see my friend, Dr. Eduardo Luque in Mexico City."

Now it was Alan's turn to be amazed. He'd wanted to get involved with Dr. Luque for years. "You know Eduardo Luque?!" ask Alan. George Rapp said that he did, picked up the phone and called him. "Eduardo, I've got this guy and he wants to talk to you." Alan got on the phone, explained Ed Simmon's spine implant issues and Dr. Luque started telling Olsen what he had designed.

Two days later, Alan Olsen was in Mexico City, scrubbing in with Dr. Luque. Remembers Alan; "Eduardo is bringing out all the implants with the screws and he gave me a mini education about sublaminar wiring, pedicle screws and plates. And I'm just eating it up and I'm just absolutely in awe of the fact I'm in the presence of Eduardo Luque. You know, the father of totally improving spine scoliosis surgical treatment from Harrington rods to sublaminar wiring."

Olsen's time with Dr. Moe in Minneapolis had shown him what happened when Harrington hooks would slide off the rods, and the pediatric patients would have to come back in for emergency surgery. "That was a big deal. Dr. Moe would be pissed as hell."

Alan had no doubt that Luque's screw and plate system would take the spinal instrumentation market by storm.

Before he left Mexico City, Dr. Luque told Alan one more thing; ""Before you do anything with this Alan, you need to go see Rich Ashman at Texas Scottish Rite Hospital, because he's doing some testing on screws and plates."

L.D. Beard and Alan had been through the experience of developing new markets for medical devices at Richards. They knew the drill, the pitfalls and the resources required.

Spine, they all agreed, could be a huge opportunity. And Luque and his inventions were the way in.

If...the FDA would approve Luque's devices.

If...Zimmer, who had a business relationship with Dr. Luque, would sign off on Biotechnology negotiating with Luque and, finally, if, somehow, they could find the resources to pay for surgeon training, salespeople and everything required to build a spinal implant business.

Alan and L.D. approached Zimmer. According to Olsen Zimmer said: "Yeah, you can make the Luque plates. You can have all his stuff. He's a total pain in the butt."

L.D. hired an FDA consultant who told him that Luque's implants looked like ordinary bone plates and screws. Which meant that they could be cleared by the FDA under Section 510(k), provided they were labeled the same way as the products in place before 1976.

"So, we filed a 510(k) as bone plates and bone screws," recalls L.D. "Of course, we were not permitted to market as anything but bone plates and bone screws. We couldn't market them as spinal products."

The first year that Danek was part of Biotechnology, the combined companies lost several hundred thousand dollars. In '86 the loss narrowed to a couple hundred thousand. In '87 Biotechnology made its first profit.

One key to this success was L.D.'s commitment to make quality products that could withstand rigorous testing procedures. He talked to Olsen about this, who in turn consulted with Dr. Luque, who said that Texas Scottish Rite Hospital in Dallas would be a good choice.

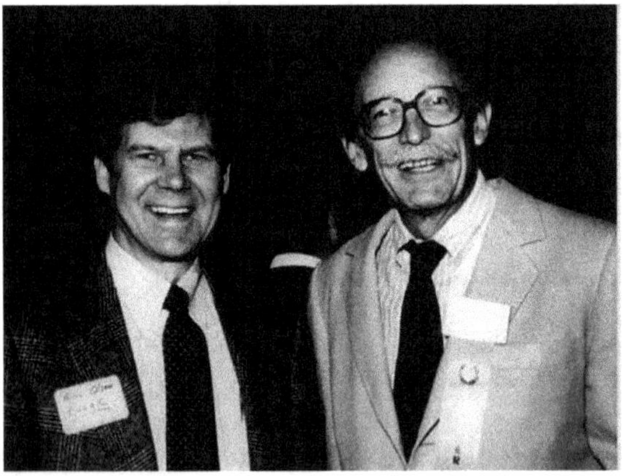

Alan Olsen and Dr. Eduardo Luque, circa 1988

A. Seth Greenwald, D.Phil.(Oxon)

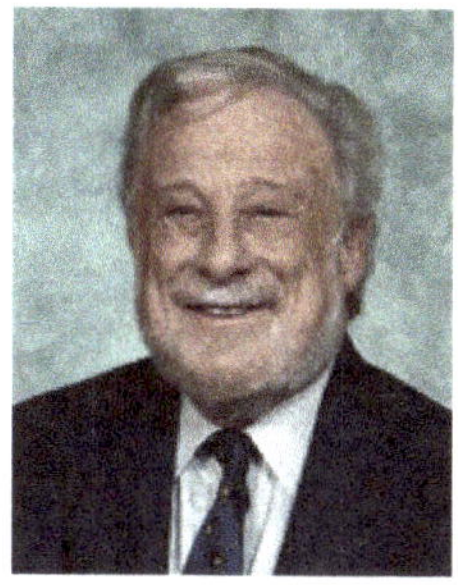

Dr. A. Seth Greenwald is currently Director of Orthopaedic Research Laboratories. He is the Founder and now, Emeritus Director, of the prestigious **Current Concepts in Joint Replacement** meetings. Dr. Greenwald received his doctorate in orthopaedic and engineering sciences from Oxford University, England in 1970 and holds advanced degrees from the Massachusetts Institute of Technology and Columbia University.

Dr. Greenwald has received many honors, notably, The American Academy of Orthopaedic Surgeons' Kappa Delta Award for outstanding orthopaedic basic science research, The Presidential Medal of the British Orthopaedic Association, The SICOT Medal for lifetime contributions to orthopaedic education and research, The Lifetime Achievement Award of the International Society for Technology in Arthroplasty (ISTA).

Dr. Greenwald still resides in Cleveland and his influence on the practice of orthopaedics can never be overstated.

Frank Janson

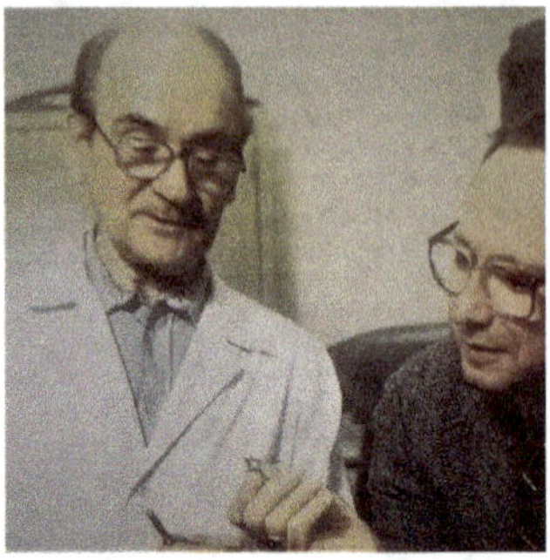

Frank Janson (left) with Art Steffee (right) Source: St. Vincent's Charity Hospital and Health Center

Born Franciszek Janik in Germany but raised in Poland, Frank entered military flight school in 1935. He escaped the invading German army, fleeing to Britain where he joined the RAF and was one of the pilots in the Battle of Britain. He was part of the 300th, 301st and 302nd squadrons. Between 1940 and 1943 he flew nonstop. For his service, he received the Distinguished Flying Medal (Britain), the Order of Virtuti Militari (Poland) and other decorations. His many contributions to medicine include advancement of kidney dialysis, thoracic and orthopedic surgery, the first total vertebral replacement and the Steffee Plate. Of the seven men from his hometown to serve in World War II, Frank was one of only two who survived. He died at age 92 in 2012 in Trinity, Florida.

CHAPTER ELEVEN: FROM COTREL TO TSRH

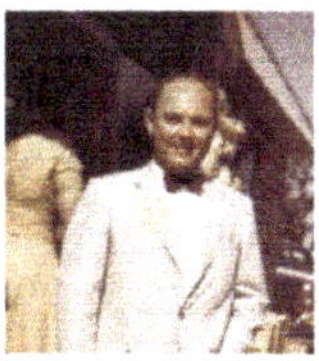

Yves Cotrel in Los Angeles, 1958

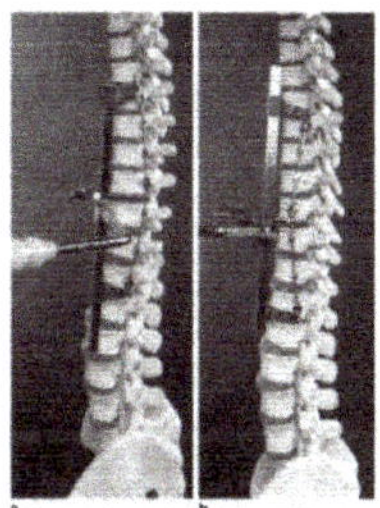

Zielke VDS System, with its characteristic 3.2mm rod

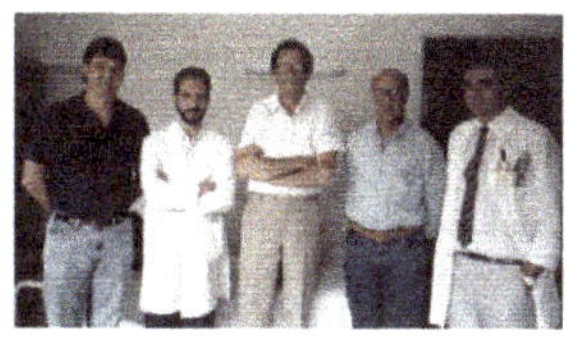

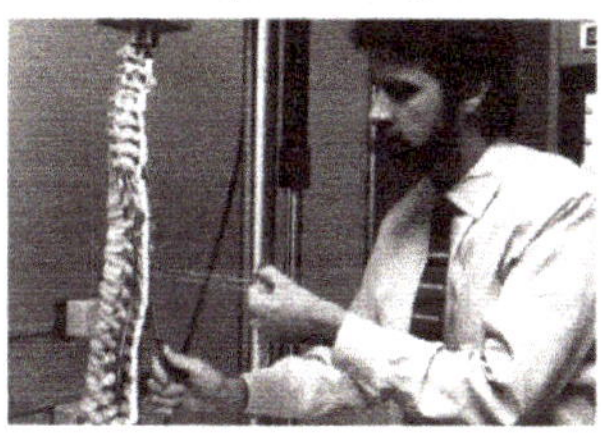

Rick Ashman, Ph.D., at TSRH circa 1990

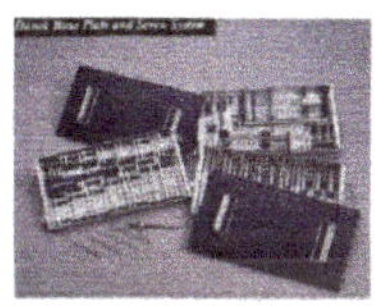

Alan Olsen (far left) with Dr. Eduardo Luque (tall man in the middle) and colleagues at Luque's Mexico City Clinic. Circa 1989

The TSRH System, circa 1990

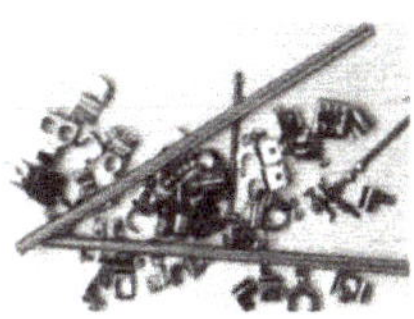

The "hardware" of spinal correction surgery circa 1990

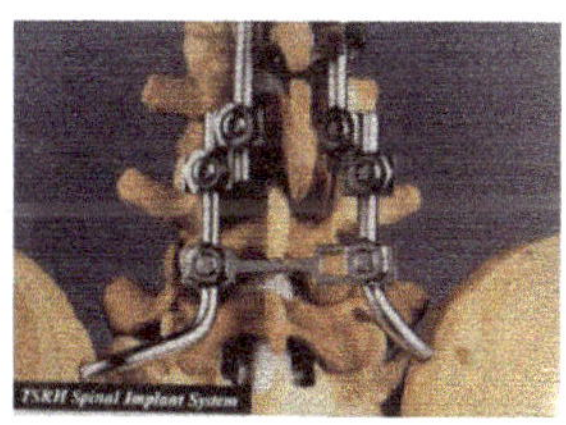

The original Danek TSRH system circa 1990

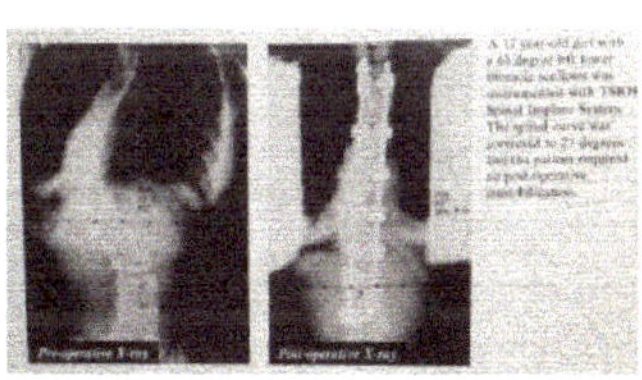

Pre and post op x-rays of the Danek TSRH system correcting severe idiopathic scoliosis. Image and description from Danek's 1991 prospectus

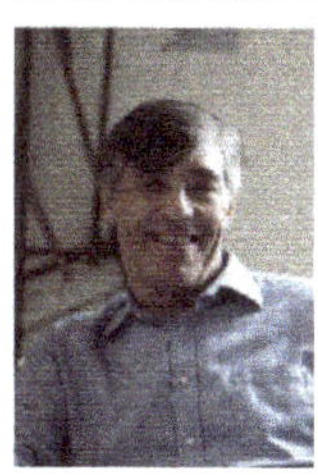

Mike Sherman

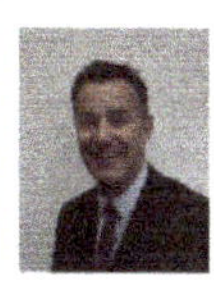

Joseph V. Lash, Danek's banker for the purchase of Sofamor

In late 1958, Yves Cotrel, a 33-year old French scoliosis physician and surgeon, embarked on a tour of the major scoliosis surgery centers in the United States and Canada. Mr. and Mrs. Richard Eaton of New York City, who were connected with the French Medical Corps during World War II, paid his way.

Cotrel started his tour at New York City's *Hospital for Ruptured and Crippled* (now Hospital for Special Surgery) at the Margaret Caspary scoliosis clinic with the legendary John R. Cobb. Cobb, who had designed and finished one of the most important studies about scoliosis and its causes, collecting data from thousands of patients—mostly poliomyelitis children—was, at the time, using a turnbuckle plaster jacket in combination with spinal fusion to treat his patients. Harrington's rod, which was in its final development stages in 1958 and was soon to be commercialized by Zimmer, was, in Cobb's view, "weird" and "completely crazy."

Cobb's foundational studies, however, which were highly accurate, have stood the test of time and remain in use today as a simple, reliable method for measuring the angle of spine curvature known as the "Cobb angle."

Cotrel's next stop was Pasadena, California, and Joe Risser. Joseph C. Risser, one of the giants upon whose shoulders Harrington, Moe, Winter, Luque and, later, Cotrel would stand on, first made his mark on spine surgery in 1936 when he and his colleagues described scoliosis's progression in untreated patients. They meticulously documented the gradual increase in deformity between the ages of 5 years and 10 years and accelerated growth and deformity between the ages of 10 years and 15 years.

Eleven years later, 1947, Risser described how spinal development and the iliac apophysis are related. By 1958, the year Cotrel visited him, a grading system based on his observations was used across the United States. Risser had, according to Cotrel, so much scoliosis knowledge and experience that he decided to extend his stay beyond the planned month.

That same year and, yes, while Cotrel was visiting, Risser gave his daughter away in marriage to a brilliant young surgeon from Mexico City, Eduardo Luque.

After Pasadena, Cotrel went to Minneapolis visiting with John Moe at the Twin Cities Spine Center. Cotrel later said of Moe, "I was immediately captivated by this large smiling giant. He wasn't dogmatic about his ideas and readily accepted those of others with curiosity, consideration, and interest—even those of a young surgeon from another country just passing through. I had rarely encountered such an open mind in my earlier experiences." As he did with Risser in California, Cotrel extended his stay in Minneapolis to learn "what was and what was not to be done."

That year, 1958, John Moe, who was a prolific writer, wrote an endorsement of facet fusion, thorough decortication, and the use of autologous bone to more reliably achieve bone fusion. He would later co-create the King-Moe classification system for adolescent idiopathic scoliosis.

Cotrel returned to the l'Institut Calot de Berck sur Mer, France, a changed surgeon.

With everything he learned rattling around in his head Dr. Cotrel created, with the help of Mr. Belembert's workshop, a system for testing, prototyping and eventually fabricating many of his ideas.

Between 1959 and 1975 Belembert's workshop grew into a manufacturer and supplier of such products as EDF plasters for early-onset scoliosis; an active preoperative continuous traction system; a spinal surgery table for perioperative correction; a tension band plating of the tibia with autologous grafting—the tension band being fixed with hooks at the ends, a dynamometric outrigger for scoliosis correction (precursor of the Harrington method); and a device for transverse traction (DTT) that was used in combination with the Harrington rod.

In 1973 the workshop was renamed Sofamor (SOciété de FAbrication de Matériaux Orthopédique) with Raoul Lanoy, better known among Sofamor employees, as "the doctor" serving as head engineer.

In 1975, at the age of 50, Cotrel suffered three cardiac arrests and retired from active surgery. Product development, through Sofamor, which now employed his daughter Doctor Marie-Hélène Plais-Cotrel, and son M. Philippe Cotrel, became his focus.

Between 1976 and 1983, in collaboration with Professor Jean Dubousset of Hôpital St. Vincent de Paul (Paris), Cotrel created a revolution in spinal deformity treatment and changed the surgical approach to spinal deformity forever. It was a set of 3D implants capable of correcting the spine in three dimensions, that we know today as the CD Instrumentation and Implant set.

In September 1985 Raymond Roy-Camille implanted the first CD with pedicle screws with Christian Mazel. In 1987 Claude Argenson was the first to use the CD in fractures.

Yves Cotrel, who had heard that Howmedica's largest distributor in the United States, Stuart Medical in Greensburg, Pennsylvania, was distributing European sourced spinal implants and instrumentation, booked a flight to Pittsburgh, about 40 miles from Greensburg, to pay Abe Glasser and Stuart Medical a visit.

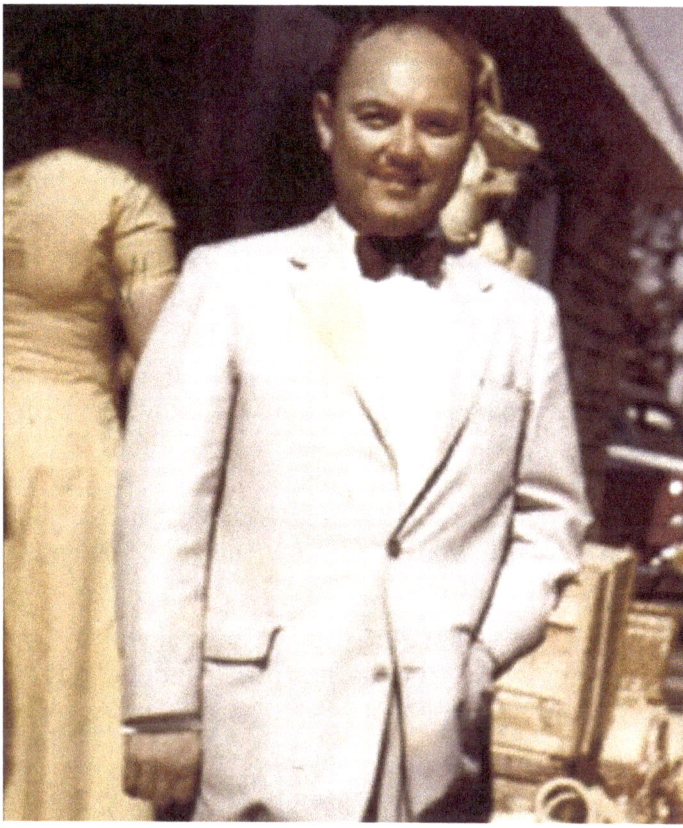

Yves Cotrel in Los Angeles, 1958

Abe Glasser, Stuart Medical and the One and Only Julius Falcon

High schooler Julius Falcon started working for Abe and Gloria Glasser's medical distribution company in 1969. He would walk over to their warehouse, work the dock, stock goods and between 1969 and 1973, through college (the legendary Slippery Rock University in Butler County, Pennsylvania) Falcon worked on and off at the Glasser's company.

Abe had been a U.S Navy pharmacist mate during World War II and, in 1951 with his wife Gloria, started Stuart Medical. He started selling band aids to Pittsburgh area hospitals. Over the years he and Gloria added literally everything a hospital could possibly need and by 1979 were employing more than 200 people in their Greensburg warehouse.

Falcon, a wrestler in high school and an athletic trainer in college who absolutely loved kinesiology, anatomy, athletic training, and all of his orthopedic courses, was working at 84 Lumber as a manager trainee when, in 1979, he stopped by Stuart Medical to chat with his long-time, on-and-off employer, Abe Glasser.

"So, Abe and I had a great conversation," remembers Julius. "He asked me, 'Julius, do you know anything about scoliosis?' I said, "Yeah, we learned about that in school. There's C shaped curves, there's S shaped curves. But you know that's just the curve from one side when you look into your body from the side, you've got a kyphosis and lordosis."

"Abe's eyes were bugging out of his head. I was throwing out terms that he had heard about, but he didn't know anything about."

There was a very specific reason Abe asked Julius that question. And that reason was John Moe, the very same surgeon who, 21 year earlier, had trained a young Yves Cotrel at the Twin Cities Spine Clinic and Fairview Hospital in Minnesota.

Doctors Moe, Robert Winter, David Bradford, and the other surgeons at the clinic were Stuart Medical customers.

Moe was stuck in U.S. Customs at La Guardia airport and had called Abe for help. Moe was returning from the Werner Wicker Kilnik in Bad Wildungen, Germany, where he was observing Klaus Zielke perform anterior spine surgery using a novel set of instruments and implants. Klaus gave Moe a set, which Moe hand-carried onto the plane. When he landed in New York and declared the spine surgery instruments and implants to U.S. customs, the agents stopped him cold.

Abe had the required licenses for importing medical devices, so he was able to pop Moe and the Zielke VDS loose.

Which is roughly when Julius Falcon providentially showed up, giving Abe an impromptu scoliosis lecture.

Abe said to Julius, “Oh you got to come down here and work with me.” And the rest, in actual fact, is spine history. Falcon came on board and would stay with Abe and Gloria’s Stuart’s Medical for the next 20 years.

Between 1979 and 1986, the largest spinal implant and instrument supplier in the world was Greensburg, Pennsylvania-based Stuart Medical—the only company selling the Zielke VDS (manufactured by ULRICH in Frankfort, Germany) and, later, Sofamor’s revolutionary Cotrel-Dubosset (CD) system in the United States.

The practice of spine surgery was beginning to find its legs.

Falcon remembers it was an intense and remarkable time in his life. “My beeper would go off, I would call in and Abe would say, ‘Julius we're going to catch a flight, we're going to Germany to watch Dr Zielke do surgery. Okay?’ And a day later, I’m sitting with Abe on that aircraft. One trip, I remember, a young kid comes walking up the aisle, introduces himself to Abe and says, ‘Are you Mr. Glasser?’ ‘Yes’. He goes, ‘Well, I'm Randy Betz, one of the doctors that's going to Germany to observe Dr Zielke doing surgery.’ Dr. Betz was 33 years old at the time.”

Randal Betz, M.D., prior professor of orthopedic surgery at Temple University School of Medicine, former Chief of Staff and Medical Director of the Spinal Cord Injury Program at Shriners Hospital for Children in Philadelphia and an internationally renowned researcher and author, remembers those early trips well.

"Abe Glasser would sponsor us to go to Germany," he recalls. "In 1986 that was my first real exposure to anterior spine surgery. In my fellowship I never saw the front of the spine. It was a real eye opener to see Zielke perform anterior spine surgery."

"Zielke was a very powerful man. No one told him anything. His staff was petrified of him. Technically, he was superb. It was an eye opener on how medicine in Europe was being practiced. Zielke himself is very gracious good thinker, very good technician."

"David Krauss from Pittsburgh, who was a well-known spine surgeon, attended the visit to Dr Zielke's clinic at the same time and when we returned Randal Betz went to Pittsburgh to do the first case using Zielke instrumentation with David Kraus. Dr Kraus in turn came to Philadelphia to assist Randal Betz with his first Zielke case."

Dr. Betz remembers that the Zielki System "Was a skinny (3.2mm) threaded rod, with a lot of nuts. Basically, it was a pedicle screw or vertebral body screw threaded rod and with these nuts. You had to rotate the nuts to move the spine along. He had a derotation device, actually a lordosing device which increased the lordosis in the spine. We know today, in 2022, that was wrong. But it worked because when you took the discs out. We didn't have good cages then, the impact of bone graft, the spine with kyphosis so trying to maintain the lordosis was actually the right thing to do. Serendipitously it worked. It was a huge advance for patients with myelodysplasia."

One of the more unique aspects of the Zielke system was that 3.2mm rod. Why 3.2mm?

The answer is John Moe. According to Falcon, "When John Moe and Klaus Zielke began their relationship, John Moe had a tremendous respect for Zielke and called Paul Harrington on the phone and said, "Paul, there's this young German doctor I want you to meet.

He really understands scoliosis and he's got a great idea here. I would love for you to meet with him, and you guys should speak about things." Zielke, with Moe's introduction, traveled to Houston, Texas, to meet John Harrington. Zielke developed so much respect for Harrington that he made his threaded rod a 3.2mm, or 1/8 of an inch, in his honor." 3.2 mm was the diameter of the Harrington compression rod used on the transverse processes.

The Zielke VDS system for anterior spine surgery was an immediate hit although Abe would not sell it unless surgeons completed training. Once "certified" by Zielke or a surgeon well versed in the system (John Moe, for example) surgeons were allowed to purchase the Zielke system for about $35,000. Abe did have loaner sets but shipped them out only on a case by case basis. That policy would later face a severe test from Memphis-based Danek Medical.

Klaus Zielke's system was a modification of a 1964 system developed by Allen Dwyer of Australia, who performed one of the first posterior releases, resecting the ligament and capsular structures overlying the facet joints on the concave side and excising any fibrous and boney ankylosis between the lamina, followed by corrective instrumentation via an anterolateral approach. Unfortunately, Dwyer's system didn't de-rotate the spine and patients experienced a high rate of late curve progression and cable fracture due to pseudarthrosis.

Zielke's innovation was a ventral derotation spondylodesis [VDS] system.

Sapporo, Japan's Kyoshi Kaneda also developed a modification of Dwyer's system which was a two-rod system to function as an anterior multi-segmental construct to treat thoracolumbar and lumbar scoliosis.

In 1976, Mexico City's Eduardo Luque developed segmental spinal instrumentation based on the principle of lateral bending as the predominant corrective force. The rods were fixed proximally and distally with sublaminar wires. After excising any contracted structures on the concave side and performing facetectomies on both sides, the wires that encircled the lamina and the rod at each segment was tightened to straighten the spine in the coronal plane.

Then came Cotrel-Dubosset.

In 1984, Yves Cotrel visited Greensburg to see Glasser. "One day, Mr. Glasser said to me, 'Julius, I have a French guy coming here. His name's Dr Cotrel. I want you to take a look at what he has,'" recalls Falcon.

Falcon was fully aware that surgeons were generally uncomfortable with the anterior surgical approach to the spine, especially on children. But, when the Zielke was indicated surgeons got the best results going anteriorly. The big medical centers at the time, Minneapolis, Chicago, New York City, Los Angeles, Philadelphia, were doing anterior spine surgery.

What Cotrel showed both Glasser and Falcon was a posterior approach which could rotate the spine using multiple hooks, different types of hooks, laminar hooks, transverse process hooks, pedicle hooks—which didn't protrude into the canal.

Falcon was very impressed. "It made great sense to me, and I thought 'Aha, well, this is going to take off.'"

"Cotrel's system didn't have a compression rod, nor a distraction rod. It had two solid rods that were seven millimeters on the OD with, including the knurls. It was a big, 7.0mm heavy thick rod and it was strong. I knew what the fear was about fracture and breakage. The Luque rod was a nice and solid 6.4mm (3/16") rod. Those didn't break. When I looked at the ability of Cotrel's design to compress and distract with multiple hooks of fixation and a safe method of connection—not a sublaminar wire—and surgeons wouldn't have to go anteriorly as much."

"The next day Abe wanted to know my thoughts, 'Julius, what did you think of that system?' I said, 'Abe, you have got to get this system.' And he got angry. 'Why?! Why?' I said, 'Because it does things nothing else does. Why don't you want it?' He goes 'Well, Dr Cotrel only wants us to make 20%.'"

Abe did sign an exclusive distribution agreement for Cotrel's system (manufactured by Sofamor). The first U.S. surgeons to use it were Dr. Kenton D. Leatherman in 1984 and Dr. Harry L. Shufflebarger in 1985.

Cotrel's system freed patients from post-operative immobilization and presented spine surgeons with a major advance in scoliosis surgery. As more surgeons were trained, it became obvious that pedicle screws were superior in achieving fixation of all three spinal columns and correcting the deformity in all three dimensions.

Alan Olsen Meets Eduardo Luque

In the latter part of 1985, Alan Olsen, founder of five-year old Danek Medical, who had just merged his company with Warsaw, Indiana-based Biotechnology, Inc. (the combined firms were named Danek Medical) was contacted by one of Biotechnology's East Coast distributors, John Agricola. A customer, Dr. Ed Simmons, was having issues with the early Zielke rod and screw spinal implants.

Olsen visited Simmons who, as Olsen recalls, starts pulling out X-rays and showing him the structural problems with Zielke's system. "Dr. Simmons was pointing to different cases, and he says, 'on this one, the screws are breaking', 'on this one, the rod is breaking'. Immediately Olsen started working on a solution, literally creating sketches on the plane ride back to see his business partners and two of Biotechnology founders, L.D. Beard and orthopedic surgeon George Rapp in Warsaw, Indiana. Rapp immediately put Olsen in touch with Eduardo Luque in Mexico City and in literally days, Olsen was scrubbing in and observing the inimitable Dr. Luque in action.

"Eduardo was bringing out all the stuff he'd been working on, sublaminar wires, pedicle screws and plates. And I'm just eating it up and I'm just absolutely in awe of the fact I'm in the presence of Eduardo Luque," remembers Olsen. "Luque is the father of totally changing scoliosis spine surgery from Harrington rods to sublaminar wiring. I scrubbed in all these scoliosis cases."

The gears in Olsen's head were spinning, which Dr. Luque could clearly see. He turned to Olsen and said, "Before you do anything with this Alan, you need to go see Rich Ashman at Texas Scottish Rite Hospital, because he's doing testing on various screws and plates."

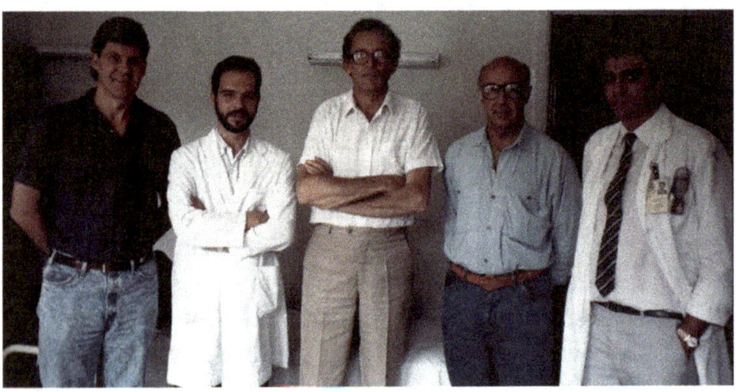

Alan Olsen (far left) with Dr. Eduardo Luque (tall man in the middle) and colleagues at Luque's Mexico City Clinic. Circa 1989

There are about 250 children's hospitals in the United States. A fair number started as "Crippled Children" hospitals and treated, at little or no cost to the family, children afflicted with poliomyelitis, cerebral palsy, spina bifida, scoliosis and other deformities of the musculoskeletal system. The Shriner's hospital system, Gillette Children's in Minnesota, the New York Hospital for Crippled Children and Memphis's St. Jude's Research Hospital are but four examples. Texas Scottish Rite Hospital had similar origins and had evolved to offer orthopedic care at no cost to families.

Rich Ashman, with a Ph.D. in biomechanical engineering from Tulane University, joined Dallas's Texas Scottish Rite Hospital (TSRH) in late 1984. Joining him in the lab were Drs. Charlie Johnston and Tony Herring. Eventually Ashman would become its hospital's Director of Research. TSRH was well known for its academic research capabilities and Ashman was joining the hospital as the revolution in spinal surgery was picking up steam.

One of his first tasks was to get an MTS Testing machine (a four-month wait). He was introduced to Mike Sherman, a Bioengineering Masters student at The University of Texas Health Science Center in Dallas and UT-Arlington. Mike had access to an Instron machine at Dallas Veterans Administration Hospital. "Charlie Johnston and I were planning a study of fatigue failure mechanisms of subliminal wiring systems." Over the next several months Rich, Mike, and Charlie used the VA's mechanical test machine.

"When I joined Charlie and Tony at Texas Scottish Rite Hospital, our overall objective was to do a deep dive into the mechanical advantages and disadvantages of the available scoliosis instrumentation systems. Our goal was not necessarily to develop a new system, but rather better understand the mechanics of the existing spine implant systems, both from the standpoint of how they could be used to better correct and stabilize deformities and avoid system failures."

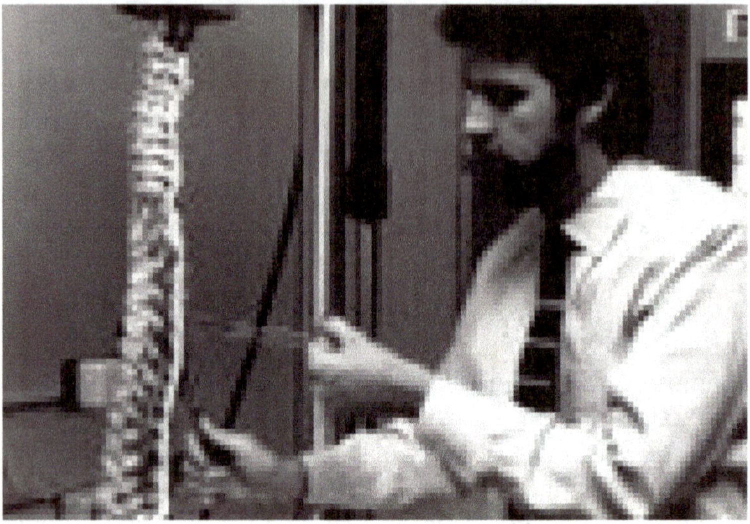

Rich Ashman, Ph.D., at TSRH circa 1990

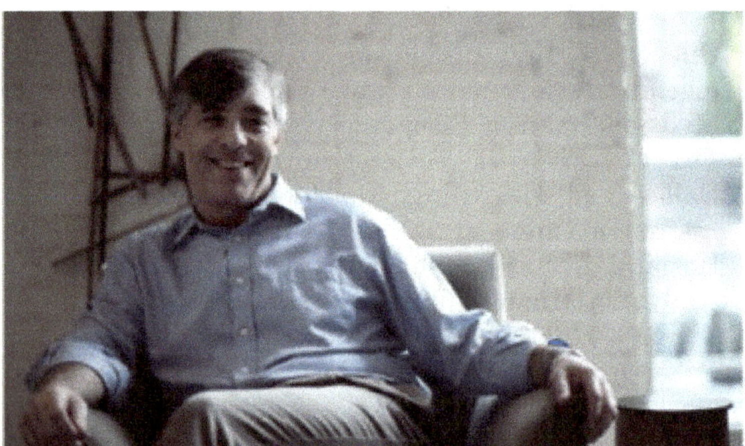

Mike Sherman

At that time the only posterior systems on the market were the Harrington and the Luque subliminal wire system. Harrington's system was increasingly being used in different ways than as first designed. Surgeons were bending and contouring the rods and using two hooks on top. They also would add subliminal wires in the center of the construct and wire the rods together. Surgeons were using combinations of Luque sublaminar wiring with Harrington rods.

These new combinations of hooks and wires on multiple vertebrae were loading the rods in ways which exacerbated the known fatigue problems of the Harrington rods. Aside from the fatigue characteristics of these hybrid systems, Ashman and Johnston were interested in how the combinations of hooks and wires affected the overall stiffness of the constructs.

Their interest in overall construct stiffness was developed years earlier when Charlie Johnston and Ashman first met in New Orleans. Ashman's biomechanical background prior to 1984 was as a faculty member at Tulane primarily studying bone mechanics and bone remodeling. "I met Charlie through Dr. Andy King at Children's Hospital in New Orleans. Charlie and I subsequently worked on a biomechanical comparison of the Zielke and Dwyer anterior spine instrumentation systems. This work was presented at the Scoliosis Research Society in 1984 and I think it was the first work using construct stiffness as a biomechanical criterion to compare spine systems."

"We believed overall construct stiffness was key to the bone fusion process. Correction of the deformity was usually primary in the surgeon's mind, but we were becoming more interested in the spine fusion process, particularly how the implant systems limited motion between vertebrae. One needs to limit motion to achieve fusion, but a construct that is too stiff can cause stress shielding of the bones and limit fusion."

By mid-1985 they had a decent understanding of the limitations of these hybrid systems and wanted to address not only the fatigue problems caused by the ratchet mechanism of the Harrington rod design, but also improve overall construct stiffness.

"At some point I really started to concentrate on more effective ways to connect rods together. The key was coming up with a connector that provided significant strength, but also small enough to implant." Sometime within 1985, Ashman came up with a clamp mechanism which would go on to be known as the Crosslink™ connector for spine rods.

Remembers Ashman, "Surgeons at Scottish Rite Hospital performed maybe 20 or so cases using the initial Crosslink connectors with Harrington and Luque rods." It was a clear improvement over wiring rods together. The TSRH team found the Crosslink connectors improved the overall stiffness and the correctability of the Harrington and Luque rod constructs both in the lab and in surgery. "At some point we began to look at hooks using the same three point shear clamp mechanism."

By 1985, a few months before Alan Olsen arrived, Ashman had the Crosslink and was exploring the idea of central hooks on a Harrington or plain rod—really to avoid Harrington's notches which, he knew, were potential fatigue points. "I was just thinking, 'Okay, we could use a plain rod, and the Crosslink connectors, have hooks that you can place up or down and have the semblance of a complete set for posterior spine correction,'" remembers Ashman. He didn't have all of the instrumentation, but he had the basic implants.

Then the Cotrel-Dubosset system, marketed by Stuart Medical, arrived in the U.S. "Several surgeons at the hospital had seen it presented at a national meeting. It was obviously a complete and well thought out system and the TSRH surgeons ordered it as soon as they could. Shortly after the surgeons at the hospital stated using the CD system. They started coming to me asking for our Crosslink with connectors sized for the larger 7mm CD rods. I had a few sets made but really needed to find someone to take on manufacturing the Crosslink."

The TSRH Crosslink was a clear improvement over Cotrel-Dubosset's DTT connector.

"I remember thinking 'Well, we had some good ideas, but it looks like these guys pretty much, you know, scooped us on whatever we were doing as far as implant development.' We weren't having any luck talking with device companies anyway. Several companies we had talked to said they wanted to get out of the spine implant market and weren't entertaining any new systems. So, I put my system into a cardboard box and stuck it on the shelf."

Then Ashman gets a call from Tony Herring saying Eduardo Luque has a new implant system with some company in Memphis; "some guy wants to come to Dallas and talk to you about implant testing."

The "guy" from Memphis was Alan Olsen from Danek.

"Alan Olsen seemed like a nice enough guy, and he had brought Eduardo's new plate and screw system which they had fabricated in Danek's Warsaw factory," remembers Ashman. "The Luque system did not lock the screws to the plate (like Steffee's system). Rather, the screws pivoted and were also cannulated."

The idea was to insert the screws down the pedicle, directed by a K wire. Ashman told Olsen that he'd be happy to test the screws, but he also told Olsen just by looking at them they'd have a fatigue problem. "The first threads near the root of the screw were started too abruptly, also the cannulation would make the screw even weaker." Ashman said the threads needed to be tapered in near the root.

"We had had other companies in and out of the lab. If something was an obvious issue, we would all express our opinions. However, I don't remember any other company treating our opinions the way Alan did. He gets on the phone to his manufacturing partner, Miles Igo, at the Biotechnology factory in Warsaw and says 'Stop the presses. We've got to redesign the screw.' Okay."

Cash was very tight at Danek at the time, but Miles stopped the presses, and they made changes.

Alan, who lived in Memphis began stopping by the TSRH lab every couple of weeks or so to see how things were going. It was 1986, during one of those visits that Ashman asked Charlie Johnston if they should show Olsen what they'd been previously working on.

"So, I pull out the cardboard box with the Crosslink and the other stuff we'd been working on; we kind of laid it out. Charlie and I talked about our concepts of how the implants would work. How the hooks could be placed up or down on plain rods and how the rods would be locked together both axially and rotationally."

Remembers Ashman, "Alan Olsen was a Marlboro smoker at the time. We were just talking away and at some point, Alan starts fumbling for his pack, tries to light up a Marlboro, this while stopping us, asking 'Wait, who have you shown this to? What is the patent status, what else is in the cardboard box.' Alan was like the worst poker player in the world."

"And Alan says, 'I would like to license all this stuff from you, okay? We'll start with the Crosslink and make that first.' It was on the market, literally, in less than 30-days after the license agreement was signed." Ashman and Olsen wrote half of the license agreement, the TSRH lawyers the other half—and it still only came to one page. Danek would manufacture and commercialize it and pay the hospital 5% royalty on net sales. No time limits. No patent requirements. That's it.

With the Crosslink and more from TSRH on the way, Danek Medical (the future Medtronic Spine) had the beginnings of a full product line for spine surgery.

Ron Pickard Leaves Richards, Joins Beard and Alan Olson at Danek

Spine surgery was not like hip surgery. A failed spine surgery was significantly more dire than a failed hip surgery. And many of the patients were children.

At the time, the only other USA spinal implant company was AcroMed, founded and run by Dr. Art Steffee. The big companies, DePuy, Biomet, Zimmer, and Stryker, were trauma, rehab, and large joint reconstruction companies. To them, spine surgery products were high risk, minimal reward opportunities and, with the exception of a small handful of products, rods or hooks, they stayed away.

Pickard never lost touch with his mentor, L.D. Beard. L.D. and Alan Olsen had combined their two struggling companies—Biotechnology and Danek—and had actually come across a product and a market that, in Olsen's opinion, could be as large as total joint replacement, maybe greater.

L.D. called Ron and, together with Alan Olsen, explained the Luque screw, sublaminar wiring, TSRH Crosslinks and how, in their judgement, it would be a significant advance in spinal implants. There was, however, a problem.

Biotechnology didn't really have the resources to put a full nationwide distribution system in place for multiple new spine devices. They could certainly manufacture them, and were selling them on a limited basis, but anything beyond required capital.

"L.D. and Alan Olsen had the vision of creating a company of substance," remembers Pickard, "but they were struggling. L.D. and I had stayed in touch and at one point, L.D. and Alan and I met, and they said, 'we don't have the resources to put this together, would Richards be willing to do a license agreement and pick up the distribution of the Luque plate and screw?'"

"I put together a proposal and presented it to my boss at Smith & Nephew (the most recent owner of Richards Medical) that we do the license agreement with Warsaw Orthopedics for the Luque System. Smith & Nephew turned it down saying, basically, that they were concerned about the liability associated with the spine. Which is understandable."

"I went to L.D. and said, 'Smith & Nephew has passed on it. but I would like to maybe discuss with you the opportunity."

Forty-two year old Ron Pickard had spent his entire 23-year career at Richards Medical (owned by Smith & Nephew by 1990) and had worked his way up the ranks, taking on virtually every job in production to become president of orthopedics.

For Pickard, the prospect of leaving Richards was a wrenching one. Alex Lukianov remembers talking with Ron just before he resigned. "We were at an offsite strategic planning meeting and Ron was running it. For whatever reason I was with him in his car, and he told me he was leaving Richards and was about to announce it. And, he said, the decision was making him sick to his stomach. He was struggling specifically with how to get his decision across to the organization."

"Ron was the guy who was really the mover and the shaker that made stuff happen. Not taking anything away from Jack Blair, but, but I would credit Ron for making orthopedics the success that it was."

Or, as Rick Treharne also remembers, "Ron was the "R" in Richards."

In August 1990, Ron Pickard officially resigned from the Richards Manufacturing division of London based Smith & Nephew to become the new president and chief operating officer of Biotechnology, which was soon renamed, Danek Medical, Inc.

Funding a Start-Up in a New Medical Specialty

In mid-1989, Danek launched the system that Rich Ashman and Charlie Johnston pulled out of a cardboard box to show Alan Olsen in 1988. The system, named TSRH (for Ashman and Johnston's employer, the Texas Scottish Rite Hospital) was a system of versatile crosslinks, specialized hooks and screws that attached to rods through locking bolts.

The year TSRH was introduced to U.S. spine surgeons, Danek's sales nearly doubled to $14.6 million. Reported profit tripled to $1.9 million.

Cash operating profit, however, was just $99,741. On top of that, Danek spent $612,000 for manufacturing equipment (an investment, which meant that the spending didn't show up on the P&L) and paid $100,000 on a Note that came due.

In 1989 Danek Group burned through $707,000—even though sales nearly doubled from $7.5 million to $14.6 million.

L.D. Beard, Alan Olsen, George Rapp, and Miles Igo had endured a fire which nearly ended the company, now they were struggling to stay solvent.

George Rapp, M.D., one of the original investors and partners with Miles Igo in Warsaw Orthopedics and also, at the time, Chief of Orthopedic Surgery at St. Vincent's Hospital in Indianapolis made the phone call to a tiny Indiana based venture fund named CID, which stood for Corporation for Innovation and Development.

The fund had raised $10 million from a group of Indiana companies, notably Eli Lilly Corporation, Ball Corporation, Cummins Engine and others to fulfill a mandate to invest in local high technology.

Robert Compton

Dr. Rapp called CID and reached a young man named Robert Compton, who'd recently joined CID from First Chicago Venture Capital. Compton was also a former student of Bill Sahlman, the legendary Harvard Business School Professor of Entrepreneurship.

"Professor Sahlman is an extraordinary guy." Remembers Compton today. "He taught entrepreneurial finance and then followed his student's career paths. Professor Sahlman has taught thousands of students who've started companies or become venture capitalists."

Compton's specialty was software. Not medicine and certainly not spine medical devices. But he was scrambling to find high technology deals in mid-1980s Indiana, so Compton agreed to meet Dr. Rapp and L.D. Beard. "I was impressed by both men," recalls Compton. "Dr. Rapp is an experienced surgeon, with an appreciation for business. What struck me about L.D. Beard was what a good listener he was. L.D. has a quiet leadership style and I thought to myself, this is someone that I would work for. Super high integrity, clearly smart and a truly likable person".

Compton then met with Alan Olsen, Danek's founder and head of sales and Miles Igo, Danek's fourth partner and head of manufacturing. One pattern that Compton saw was how well each person's skill complemented the other person. Olsen was a really excellent salesman and had great rapport with surgeons. L.D. was the strong leader with well-honed management skills. Dr. Rapp brought medical expertise and Igo knew manufacturing.

A Million Dollars for...Hardware?

The Danek team asked for a million dollars—a lot for the small CID fund. Compton and his partners were thinking more like $500,000. And that, in turn, reinforced in Compton's mind the need to pull in other investors—not only to support Danek's funding needs, but also to get another set of eyes and smarts on this truly (in the late 1980s) unique business concept—selling spine surgery implants!

"I took the TSRH system out to Silicon Valley and showed it to one of the oldest and most successful venture firms in the valley." One of Compton's Harvard classmates was a junior partner there. "I went to Sandhill Road and through my friend, got a meeting with the senior partner."

Sandhill Road is arguably the birthplace of venture capital for the integrated circuit based high-tech revolution. Microsoft, Amazon, Twitter, Facebook, Instagram, and thousands of other legendary high technology companies were funded by venture firms on Sandhill Road.

Compton was at the citadel of high tech to make the Danek pitch. He handed the senior partner of this Sandhill Road venture firms Danek's system of metal rods, screws and hooks. To this day, Compton vividly remembers what happened next. "After about 10 minutes into my talk, he said, stop, stop. I could buy this stuff at a hardware store.' And he tossed it back at me. I was crushed."

His first meeting ended the trip. Sandhill Road venture firms shared information and Compton knew this particular "no", coming so swiftly and definitively, was the end of his trip.

When he got back to Indiana, Compton put in a call to Dane Miller, the founder of Biomet and one of the most savvy orthopedic executives in the industry. Dane told

Compton that he knew Danek but, reflecting the common wisdom among the large orthopedics companies like Stryker, Zimmer or DePuy, he told Compton spine surgery was dangerous—not only for manufacturers, but certainly for investors.

"I came back to my office at CID and thought, you know, I've talked to a venture capitalist who doesn't get it. I've talked to someone in the industry who says it's too risky, but I haven't talked to a customer. So, I came back to Indianapolis and scrubbed in with a really, really seasoned trauma surgeon who also did scoliosis surgery."

That surgeon was Dr. Terry Trammell, who wrote a book about putting Indy 500 drivers back together after they'd crashed. He's also done his spine fellowship with Dr. Edward Simmons in Buffalo, New York—the very same Ed Simmons who set Alan Olsen down the path of moving Danek into the spinal implant business.

"I scrubbed in and watched him do a surgery. Afterwards we sat down for coffee. I asked him, 'what do you think of spinal implant products? And what do you specifically think of the TSRH spinal implant system? He said, 'Bob, this is gonna revolutionize spinal surgery.'"

"I went back to my partners at CID, and I said, the smartest guy in Silicon Valley turned me down, Dane Miller said it was scary, but the surgeon who is the person who is ultimately going to make the buying decision, thinks this is revolutionary."

CID did the whole million dollars. And Bob Compton joined Danek's board of directors.

Danek ended 1989 with effectively three days of cash in the bank ($80,682). And were able to pay for new equipment and set the stage to sell $25 million of products in 1990—the year Ron Pickard became Danek's president and future CEO.

Back at Smith & Nephew, Pickard's departure caused many other employees to think about their own tenure. "When Ron left in late 1990, it sent ripples through the company," remembers Mike Sherman, a member of the engineering staff at Smith & Nephew. "Ron was born and raised at Richards."

One of the first to follow Pickard was Richard Treharne, Ph,D,, Smith & Nephew's Technical Manager, who joined Danek in November 1990.

Pickard took a 40% pay cut to join Danek. As he soon discovered, however, Danek had cash issues. "My first paycheck at Danek bounced. My wife called me and said, 'you remember that little old check you gave me?' I said 'yeah'. She said, 'well, the bank just called, and it isn't any good.'"

31-year old Mark Merrill, Danek's accountant at the time, moved money around to cover his new president's inaugural paycheck. Danek was not Richards, where the senior executives were judged based on the P&L (profit and loss financial statement). At his new firm, Pickard realized, cash was king. The P&L didn't pay the bills, the checking account did.

There is an old saying, start-up companies need to squeeze the nickel until the buffalo shits. Danek's executives, by and large, were in Memphis, but manufacturing was in Warsaw, Indiana. To save money, all Memphis executives drove 11 hours to get to their production plant. Remembers Pickard, "I'd leave at 4 o'clock in the afternoon and drive all night and get there the next day. But you do what you gotta do."

And yet, despite all that, Pickard, as he recalls these decades later: "I'll be honest with you. I don't think myself or anyone else at that little, tiny company...it never, ever crossed our mind that we might fail."

"Any time you start a company or any time you're in a small company like that, you have two exit strategies. You either sell it to a bigger company or you take it public," remembers L.D. Beard. "That's the way you get your investment out of it. So, I had always thought that, probably, if you're prepared to go public, then you're prepared to sell or do anything else. Because, again, everything is open and above board. You're doing financial statements. Your financial statements are public records. So, I told Alan, Miles, and Ron early on, we'll just pretend that we're a publicly owned company. Then if we want to sell to somebody, we're prepared for it. Or if we want to go public, we'll be prepared for it. The company was operated like that from 1985 forward."

Before Pickard's first month was done, he, L.D., and the entire senior management team and board of directors decided to formally begin the process of going public. Two underwriters were selected; New York-based Smith Barney, Harris Upham & Co. (lead underwriter) and Memphis-based Morgan Keegan & Company.

L.D. Beard recruited a new chief financial officer, 53-year old Gary Light, formerly the CFO for Mayflower Transit and before that partner at Arthur Anderson.

Gary Light was, in L.D.'s opinion, "a financial wizard."

Of all Danek's senior management, only Gary Light had experience with the public stock offering process. A key element, of which, was the "road show," which consists of a series of presentations on behalf of a company doing an initial public offering. The idea is to generate interest on the part of potential investors and financial analysts.

Light suggested that Pickard, who was sixteen years younger than L.D., would represent the young company better than either one of them. L.D. quickly agreed and spoke to Pickard, a conversation the latter would well remember:

"In April of '91, L.D. said, 'Look, I'm probably not going to be the person to take this company over the next number of years. If we're going to go public those who are going to be looking at this company need to be looking at the people that are going to be more actively involved in management, and therefore I think you should be chief executive officer. Because you're eventually going to be there anyway, and it would be a more fair and honest presentation of management of the company, when you're selling the company to shareholders, to represent it in that way.'"

So, the plan was, just before embarking on the IPO process, Pickard would be elected CEO and L.D. would be chairman of the board.

Then, as Pickard recalls, in late August 1990, "L.D. walked in my office and said, 'What do you think?' and I said, 'I think we're ready to launch the IPO.' L.D. said, 'No, I'm talking about the damn invasion.'" Iraq had invaded Kuwait the U.S. was mobilizing to respond and Wall Street had essentially stopped public capital raising activities.

The Nine Month IPO Delay

"I think that delay definitely worked," remembers Compton. "It didn't feel like a good thing at the time, but that delay allowed Ron and L.D. to build out the team, the intellectual property and get more systems in place."

"I was somewhat relieved," Pickard recalls. "We had more breathing room and I was trying to put an organization together, hiring and recruiting people. Doing that initial public offering, well, that was my first time. The pause wasn't a bad thing for me."

With the extra time, Pickard put together a manual detailing how Danek should be organized, which jobs needed to be filled and job descriptions. L.D. and the board approved it. Sales were doubling yet again so cash, while still tight, was steadily flowing in.

Among the people Pickard hired during the IPO delay was a young 29-year old engineer from Smith & Nephew who, as it turned out, was good friends with Rich Ashman, Charlie Johnston, and Tony Herring, the engineering and spine surgeon team that developed the TSRH spinal system—Mike Sherman. Eventually, Sherman would file more than 120 spinal implant patents for products he invented or co-invented—the most ever for a Medtronic Spine employee at that time.

In December 1990, curious about what was going on, Sherman arranged to come by and see Alan Olsen and Ron Pickard. After exchanging pleasantries, Mike was dished off to John Pafford. "So, I walk into John's office, and he says 'Uh, this is my first day. Do you have a resume?' I said, 'No, I don't have a resume.' Because I wasn't looking for a job," remembers Mike.

"We had this great conversation. I didn't know John, but he'd been in Memphis working for Wright Medical for ten years. John was impressive, he had started at Wright Medical as a drafter when he was in High School. He'd worked his way through college while he was at Wright Medical ultimately running the customs and special operation there. I went back to talk with Alan and Ron, and they said, 'Do you have any questions?' That was pretty much it and they offered me a job at Danek. I never asked them about benefits. It was a start-up. I was single. It never occurred to me that this was a risky move."

Mike wasn't due to start at Danek for another four weeks, but events were moving fast. "I rushed back to Smith & Nephew to resign. David Brumfield was my boss at the time. When I told him I was resigning, he told me he was resigning as well and that he'd have to resign to his boss, Michael DeMane, for the both of us.

Of course, several years later, Michael DeMane would join the Sofamor Danek team as well."

Also, that January, 35-year old Alex Lukianov gave his notice at Smith & Nephew and made the two-mile drive down Airways Boulevard to Danek.

The company was taking shape.

"The Spine Specialist"

Warsaw Orthopedics (renamed Danek Manufacturing) was, if nothing else, versatile. It could make soft goods. Grind metal. And, even, make replacement parts for outboard gas motors. Miles Igo, its president, could make just about anything.

But there was a price to pay for such versatility. One of Pickard's initiatives at Danek, was to coin the tagline; "The Spine Specialist" which had the effect of focusing Danek's manufacturing and product development strictly on spine.

"Ron brought a sharp, very sharp focus on spine," which Danek's culture at the time, young and increasingly dynamic, needed, remembers Compton.

The Harrington and Luque rods were antiquated. Sofamor's Cotrel-Dubosset system (distributed by Stuart Medical), the Zielke anterior system (also sold by Stuart Medical), Danek's Luque spine plate and screw system, TSRH spinal system, AcroMed's Steffee spine plate and screw—all represented a revolution in spine care. The team at Danek felt the thrill of open field running. Everything seemed possible.

By early 1991, the Danek's IPO was back on, and, Ron Pickard, Danek's new CEO, along with Gary Light, Danek's CFO introduced their rapidly growing spinal implant and instrument company to investors.

"Wall Street dramatically underestimated Ron," remembered Compton. "There was a kind of a bias against Southern companies. He was so much smarter than all of them put together. Wall Street thought they knew him. They didn't. Ron is brilliant. He was able to see way into the future and then make those remarkable decisions."

On May 17, 1991, exactly seven years after the business almost went up in flames at the Warsaw manufacturing plant, Danek raised $27 million before underwriter and legal fees and started trading on NASDAQ at $15.00 share. The public owned 22% of the company, employees and founders of the company owned 55%, CID owned 16% and Eduardo Luque owned 7%. CID's $1 million investment had grown to $20 million in less than two years.

Finally, remembers Pickard, "We were really strict about one thing. We never, ever talked about the stock market, never talked about the price of our stock. It was something that was never discussed. We always had the opinion that the stock price would take care of itself if we took care of our customers. I always said, 'Our stock goes down when we meet or exceed expectations and goes up when we fail to meet expectations.'"

Buying Yves Cotrel's Sofamor

By 1992, relations between Yves Cotrel's Sofamor manufacturing operation in France and its U.S. distributor, Stuart Medical, were increasingly strained. More than once, sales meetings between the French supplier Sofamor and its owner and inventor of the Cotrel-Dubosset system, Yves Cotrel, would devolve into shouting matches with Abe Glasser or his sales force.

Shawn McGuinn, one of Stuart Medical's sales executives remembers "We were selling the DTT, Device for Transverse Traction, from Sofamor. It was a crosslink developed by Dr. Cotrel and Dr. Dubousset. The physicians in the United States thought it was wimpy. It didn't do what it needed to do. Abe told Yves Cotrel and it became very controversial."

Mike Sherman remembers when Cotrel would lecture at Texas Scottish Rite and surgeons would raise the issue about the flimsy construction of the DTT and Dr. Cotrel would say 'It wasn't designed to be a stabilizer. It was only meant to keep the rods spread apart.'"

But, as Mike Sherman remembers, "At the end of the day surgeons needed a more stout crosslink."

Rich Ashman, Charlie Johnston, and Tony Herring developed exactly that device. They even showed it to Cotrel but, again, he said 'our crosslink is fine.'

Danek licensed the TSRH crosslink (branded the Danek Crosslink). That, along with Luque's plate and screw, were Danek's first significant spinal implant products.

At some point in 1992, word filtered to Alan Olsen and Ron Pickard that Sofamor was being shopped to potential corporate buyers. Piper, which was Sofamor's investment banker and had the sales book, was speaking to all comers—except Danek. Despite numerous requests, the Piper bankers refused to let Danek into the bidding.

It all came to a head at the 7th annual meeting of the North American Spine Society in Boston in 1992. As Alan Olsen remembers, "The bankers for Sofamor, Piper Jaffray, wouldn't give us the book. I said to Ron, 'Well, let's try and get ahold of Dr. Cotrel,' because I had just spoken to him at a poster exhibit and found out he was on his way back to France tomorrow. So, Ron and I hustled right over to his hotel. And Ron gave his pitch."

Pickard recalls that Zimmer was doing due diligence on Sofamor and were far enough along to be putting numbers to paper. "My pitch to Dr. Cotrel," said Pickard, "was 'You can certainly join Zimmer. They're going to hire a product manager to run your company and you really won't have much to say about it. Or it's gonna be run by a product manager reporting to somebody else who's reporting to somebody else who's reporting to somebody else.'"

"'Or you can join Danek, and you'll have a seat on the board. We're a public company. We have a liquid currency, and you can have a continued involvement—a say in how the company is run.' I think that pitch set well with him. As a result, we signed the necessary papers to get started."

The Sofamor Deal Goes on Life Support – Twice

Merrill Lynch was the banker representing Danek and Piper Jaffray was representing Sofamor. Ron got a call late in the afternoon before a flight to France to complete the final stage of negotiation. Merrill Lynch, his banker, was calling. They wanted to drop out. For some unspoken reason, they could no longer represent Danek.

"Oh my gosh. I was livid," remembers Pickard, "I actually yelled in the phone at this guy, the head of healthcare banking for Merrill Lynch. They were bailing out. After I hung up I remembered Joe Lash with Kidder Peabody, which at the time was owned by GE Capital."

"I'd met Joe a couple times and he and I always hit it off quite well. So, I ran Joe down that evening, and I told him the whole story. He said, 'We will be there this evening.' We spent most of that night just going over where we were, where we'd been."

When Pickard and L.D. Beard left for Paris the next day, they had new bankers and lawyers from Sherman and Sterling. The team spent three days outside of Brittany hammering out merger details.

The near-final documents were in Memphis by April 1993.

Then Dr. Cotrel called Pickard and said: 'We can't take your [Danek] stock.

"What do you mean?" Pickard asked. What it boiled down to was that Dr. Cotrel's uncle, who owned a small percent of Sofamor, would not accept Danek equity for his Sofamor equity. He wanted cash.

Pickard didn't skip a beat. "It wasn't anything we could not deal with. But, our attorneys, Sherman and Sterling, realized that this opened up a new, favorable accounting option for Danek. They told Pickard that Danek could treat the payment as Goodwill. They said, "We can create a tax situation where you can amortize Goodwill for the next six or seven years, which basically results in Danek paying no taxes."

Sherman and Sterling more than paid for themselves with that insight.

"A few years later," Pickard remembers, "the IRS showed up and said they were auditing us over the Sofamor transaction. They spent almost a year with IRS agents in the building. They left. I think, exactly 11 months after they arrived. Nothing was wrong. We did everything by the book. They closed the case."

Whose Name Goes First?

It was nearly June when Dr. Cotrel called Pickard again and said, 'I need to meet with you. Can you fly to New York?' "Absolutely," said Pickard. "We met at the Pierre Hotel in New York in Dr. Cotrel's room. He had a little cup of coffee in his hands. His hands were shaking, and the coffee was splattering out of the cup. And I said; 'What's wrong, Dr. Cotrel?' And he says; 'I cannot do the deal.' I said: 'But we've already done the deal. I mean, it's done.'"

'No, no, no, I can't do the deal.' And I said: "So what happened?" And he said: 'Your company is buying my company. I know that. But you will have your name first. And I, I, I cannot do that.'"

"So, I said; 'You're telling me that we're going to cancel this whole deal because putting Danek's name first and Sofamor next is impossible.' And Dr. Cotrel said; 'Yes. I know you would never agree to anything else.'"

"I said: 'Why don't we call the company Sofamor Danek?' And Dr. Cotrel literally stood up and hugged my neck. I felt strange sitting in this hotel room with a little old Frenchman hugging my neck."

"I agreed to the name change and, on the way, back to Memphis, I thought to myself, you know, I just committed to something that I'm not sure how the board of director's is gonna react." In fact, it took about one second after Pickard described his meeting with Dr. Cotrel for the board to agree to the name change.

"I had no reason for any concern. It was a nonissue at the board. But it meant a tremendous amount to Dr. Cotrel and his entire family. It really solidified a relationship that lasted all the way up until he passed away."

"Even today with his daughter Marie-Helene Plais, M.D., who was clearly the apple of his eye and very active in the management of the company. I've gotten a number of handwritten notes from Dr. Cotrel over the years expressing his support for me and everything the company wanted to do."

Danek purchased Sofamor in June 1993 for approximately 6 million shares or 25% of the combined company's equity. Six years later, Sofamor Danek was sold to Medtronic $3.7 billion of which approximately $925 million went to the Cotrel family.

The End of Spine at Stuart Medical

Once Danek's purchase of Sofamor was official, Stuart Medical's rights to distribute Sofamor products transferred to the newly named Sofamor Danek, based in Memphis, Tennessee. That same year Abe Glasser sold Stuart Medical to a Pittsburgh investor; Henry

Hillman who folded Stuart Medical into North American Medical. Finally, in July 1999, Owens and Minor purchased Stuart Medical from the Henry Hillman Family for $155 million.

The Effect of Sofamor on Danek

In 1994, the first full year with Sofamor, combined company's sales reached $162 million (of which the Cotrel-Dubousset line of products accounted for 30%), reported net profit was $24 million and cash in the bank stood at $13 million.

Acquiring Sofamor brought distribution in 24 new countries to Danek. It added the CD Spine System which was designed primarily to treat thoracic and lumbar spinal deformities and fractures to Danek's portfolio. Later came the Compact Cotrel-Dubousset system (CCD) which was sold to treat degenerative spine disc disease of the lumbar and sacral spine. Then came the CD Horizon™ system which introduced new types of hooks and screws and brought an increased level of versatility to surgeons.

Likewise, the TSRH system continued to evolve with the Variable Angle Screw, Central Post Hook, Lateral Offset Plate, Open Eyebolt, and Top Tightening components. All of which, gave surgeons new capabilities including interchangeability of components which improved ease of use for spine surgeons.

This Danek team, as we will describe in upcoming articles, would come to define Modern Spine Surgery is several astonishing ways:

- Invent and bring to market the first surgical navigation system (Stealth Station)
- Invent and bring to market the first minimally invasive pedicle screw instrumentation system (Sextant System developed by Mike Sherman and Kevin Foley, M.D., which was built off of the CD Horizon platform)

- Bring through the FDA and ultimately to market the first bone morphogenic protein.

And then, of course, there is the role Ron Pickard and the Danek senior management played in literally saving Modern Spine Surgery during pedicle screw litigation and the related FDA firestorm.

Safe Medical Devices Act of 1990

Even as the steps to go public were underway, there was a new item that had to be addressed, not just by Sofamor Danek but by every orthopedic implant manufacturer: Congress had enacted the Safe Medical Devices Act of 1990, which increased the FDA's authority to regulate medical devices, including implants. The law took effect the following year, and the reach of the new regulations was extensive, imposing new requirements not only on manufacturers, but hospitals and other health care facilities as well. Specifically, if the facility becomes aware of any serious health problems ("adverse events") experienced by a patient and the problems appear to be related to a medical device, it must be reported both to the manufacturer and to the FDA.

A manufacturer of a device that is "substantially equivalent to a Class III device" (under defined by the Medical Device Amendments of 1976) must also certify to the FDA that it has completed a thorough search for information related to the "safety and effectiveness" of that device. There is a further reporting requirement of "any correction or removal of a device, other than for routine servicing, if the action was undertaken to: (1) reduce a risk to health; or (2) remedy a violation of this Act caused by the device which may present a risk to health."

Moreover, many new high-risk devices must have extensive post-market scrutiny, meaning that manufacturers and distributors of medical devices are required to track the use of those devices by patients.

This meant that Danek would have to develop "a method of device tracking" and annually certify the number of reports it has received. This latter provision became effective in 1993.

CHAPTER TWELVE: 1993 – BEST OF TIMES AND WORST OF TIMES

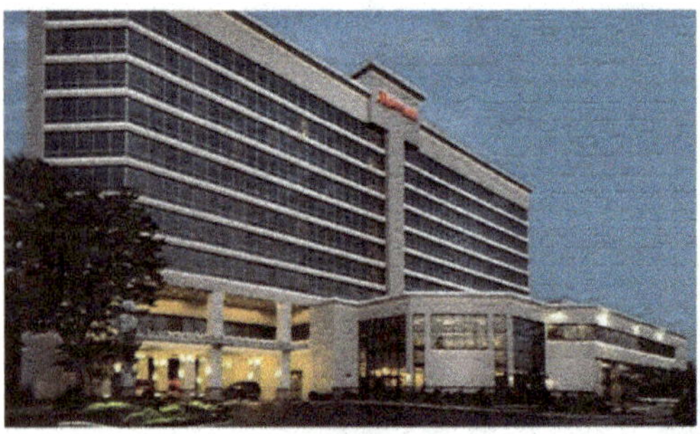

Memphis Marriott Hotel

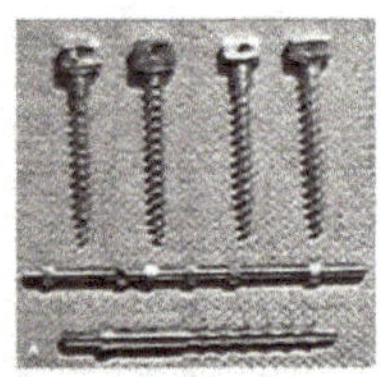

Early examples of pedicle screws and plates: Kostuik / Harrington Screws

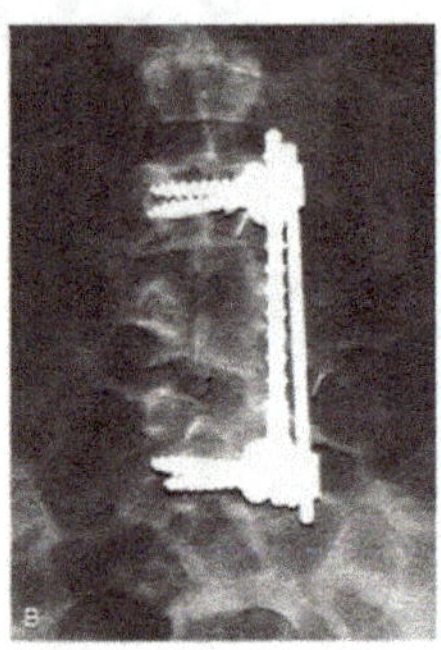

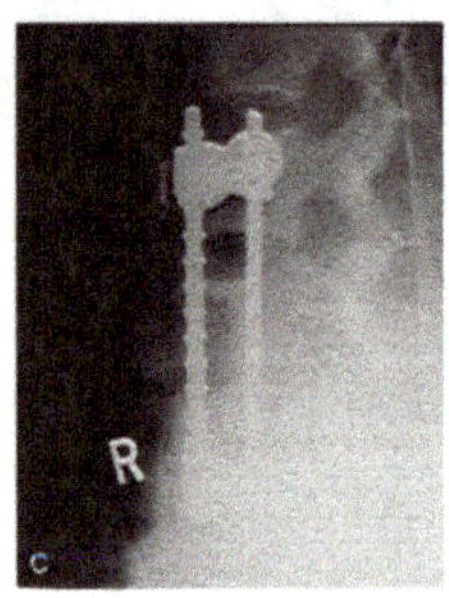

In December 1993, Sofamor Danek Group, Inc., was closing out an exceptionally good year. The company had nearly doubled in size the previous June when it acquired French orthopedic company Sofamor S.A.—staff and management were still getting used to their company's new name and its first-time listing on the New York Stock Exchange—and the future looked unbelievably bright.

Demand for hip, knee, and spinal implant devices was continuing to increase at a dizzying rate, and the company's normal inventory had quadrupled since 1991 just to keep up with orders. During the same two-year period, Sofamor Danek's net sales had jumped from just under $75 million to nearly $162 million.

True, Ron Pickard was a relatively new president and CEO, but he was cast in the same mold as the company's first CEO, L.D. Beard. The similarity between the two men was no coincidence. Both had spent their formative managerial career at Memphis's Richards Manufacturing—each had worked his way up from the bottom rungs at Richards to company president—and Beard had been instrumental in Pickard's selection as vice president of manufacturing there.

Years later, when Beard had needed a chief operating officer for his own company, he knew exactly the man he wanted, and Pickard had jumped at the chance, primarily to work with his mentor. That was in 1990, and Pickard had rapidly moved up to company CEO.

Yet even now, despite heading a major orthopedic company, Pickard still called the board chairman "Mr. Beard," a habit that would not change until both men retired. No doubt part of his deference was the age difference—Beard was sixteen years Pickard's senior—but most of it was their history together at Richards. Beard had been a top manager there while Pickard was still cleaning floors. Beard would later joke, "He tells people that he's known me since 1967, but I'd only known him since 1972. That's about right."

At Sofamor Danek they made a formidable team and usually saw eye to eye on major issues. Together they had overseen Danek's first public offering, on the NASDAQ in 1991, and now they had brought about the merger with Sofamor S.A. and moved the corporation to the Big Board. In short, they had good reason to celebrate at the annual Christmas party.

This company-wide event carried over a tradition that Beard had brought with him from Richards. It was a modest but sincere effort to reward employees and to maintain a sense of "family" among the staff despite the company's rapid growth. To make the occasion a bit more special, the affair was always held away from the company offices, usually at an upscale hotel in the Memphis area. The actual location might change from year to year, but the basic structure remained the same: an evening "dress-up" party and dance attended by employees and their spouses or dates, along with top management and their spouses.

In most ways, the 1993 party was typical. The company rented a ballroom at the Marriott Hotel in southeast Memphis, and secretaries and staff from customer service took care of the decorations. Silver foil streamers were hung from the ceiling, brightly colored cloths were placed on the tables, and a bar (wine and beer only) was set up. A disk jockey with a turntable and amplifier provided the music. But in another sense, not known to most of the employees, this particular Christmas party would be anything but typical.

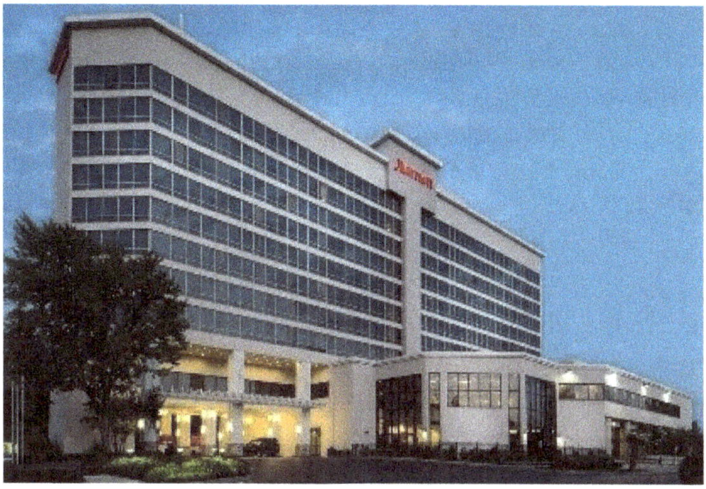

Memphis Marriott Hotel

A Public Attack on Fixation Screws in Spine Surgery

Pickard and other senior staff were aware of a potential, but minor, public relations problem. They had learned that *20/20*, a long-running ABC television "news magazine," was working on a segment about the inappropriate surgical use of spinal bone screws manufactured by AcroMed, a Cleveland orthopedic implant manufacturer. Some weeks earlier an ABC affiliate in Los Angeles had run a brief story about health problems associated with these screws, but that had not attracted much attention.

However, ABC News had now picked up on recent newspaper accounts in New Orleans about Louisiana lawsuits that alleged misuse of bone screws by doctors in spinal surgery, and *20/20* was reportedly preparing a major story about the litigation and the use of spinal screws in general. Beyond that, Sofamor Danek executives knew nothing about the upcoming program except that it was scheduled to air on December 17, 1993, the same night as the Christmas party.

Not that they were particularly concerned. No one from

20/20 had contacted the company, and there was no reason to expect a negative report even if Sofamor Danek were to be mentioned. But at the same time, it was not the kind of attention the company wanted, and those at the senior management were understandably apprehensive.

Like AcroMed, Sofamor Danek manufactured bone screws, with full Food and Drug Administration knowledge about their use in general. The previous August the FDA had sent letters to Sofamor Danek along with six other companies, cautioning them to avoid any reference in their promotional literature to "medical education programs" that might appear to encourage the use of these screws in *spinal* surgery—a procedure which did not yet have FDA clearance.

In fact, Sofamor Danek had never recommended the use of its bone screws in spinal surgery, and it considered itself in full compliance with both the FDA letter and FDA regulations.

On the other hand, nothing prevented surgeons from using any devices "off-label" if they deemed them medically appropriate for the health of their patients. It was always possible that this might occur with Sofamor Danek products as well, but the notion that a manufacturer should be considered responsible for a doctor's own independent medical judgment seemed a stretch.

Nonetheless, it was certainly a situation worth monitoring, and Pickard had quietly reserved a suite at the Marriot, one with a large-screen television so that he and other members of senior management could view the program. Eight or ten would probably want to watch the broadcast, and he did not want everyone "huddled down" in a little room trying to see and hear what was going on. Always careful with company funds, he persuaded the hotel to "comp" the suite.

The weather in Memphis on December 17 was mild,

reaching 55 degrees by mid-afternoon, and the Christmas party began as planned at seven o'clock. Besides the beer and wine, there were "heavy" hors-d'oeuvres, and very quickly the attendees—some 100-125 in all—were having a great time.

The *20/20* telecast would not start until nine o'clock, so there was plenty of opportunity beforehand to mingle and celebrate. Of course, those who knew about the program and the reserved suite kept an eye on the time and beginning about a half hour before airtime they began to quietly leave the ballroom—"snuck out," Pickard would later say. One by one they made their way to the suite; Pickard having reminded them to make sure they did not all leave at the same time.

At least one departure was not without irony: years later Pickard would still remember the song being played as he headed out the ballroom door: Elvis Presley's version of "Blue Christmas."

Those who arrived at the suite early were able to watch the last few minutes of "Hangin' with Mr. Cooper," an ABC sit-com about a high school gym coach. But soon enough—in fact, it was *20/20*'s lead story—an off-screen announcer was promising "a shocking exposé" about a surgical technique that had ruined the lives of many people. Moments later ABC News' medical editor Dr. Timothy Johnson began his report on Lake Charles, Louisiana, patients who had undergone spinal surgery and "ended up with canes and braces and ruined lives after screws and plates were implanted in their backs." The reason, he said, was because "the screws that were supposed to help them, broke."

A series of patients then described their suffering in on-screen interviews. "[I]t felt like somebody had a knife in my back." "My back felt like it was being pulled apart." "I put my wife and child through hell every day, every day, because of this." "Sometimes a leg will go out and I would fall." Others spoke of terrible pain and embarrassment in heartbreaking stories, all of which

Dr. Johnson attributed to the improper use of orthopedic screws.

The program also featured short interviews with FDA commissioner Dr. David Kessler, with medical sales personnel, with surgeons, and with the creator of the surgical technique that used the bone screws. Accusations and denials swirled back and forth.

Both the content and the thrust of the report struck the Sofamor Danek men as one-sided and manifestly unfair. They knew that many of the patients interviewed surely had chosen to undergo risky spinal surgery precisely because they were already experiencing excruciating and intractable pain. They also knew that no doctor would ever, nor could ever, guarantee that any spinal surgery would be fully successful or that it was free of all risk.

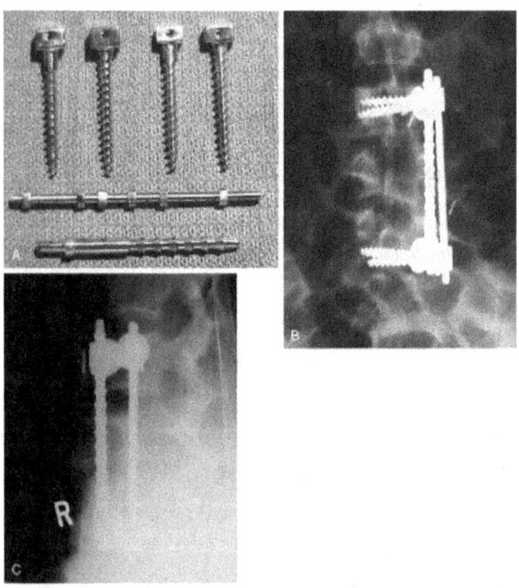

Early examples of pedicle screws and plates: Kostuik / Harrington Screws / Source: https://clinicalgate.com

But *20/20*'s account was particularly galling for another reason: it concluded that the fault lay not only with the surgeons' alleged misuse of the screws but with the manufacturers themselves. The unmistakable implication was that manufacturers were actively and wrongfully, perhaps even recklessly, promoting the use of bone screws in spinal surgery. Those who were watching the program in the Marriot suite knew otherwise, at least with regard to Sofamor Danek, and the *20/20* account had them shaking their heads. "Poor AcroMed" was the sentiment voiced most often, and Pickard believed the feeling was sincere: "We didn't say that in a mean way. It was 'How terrible it was' because we knew that what they had portrayed in the show was totally wrong."

Even so, when the segment finally ended everyone felt a sense of relief. Not one allegation had been directed specifically at Sofamor Danek. Nor for that matter had the company even been mentioned by name, although *20/20* had briefly displayed an image of a Sofamor Danek booth at an orthopedic convention. It was AcroMed and the doctor who had helped create the device that were the main targets of the piece, and they had already been sued. In contrast, Sofamor Danek had been named a defendant in a lawsuit only once in its history, and that litigation had not involved implants at all.

But it was relief constrained by caution, and Pickard remembers sharing with Beard his own uncertainty, "I don't know whether it's going to lead to anything or not."

At any rate, this was clearly not the place to speculate on what might or might not happen. Now much less anxious—at least the uncertainty was over—the group rejoined the celebration, which broke up around eleven o'clock.

In the days immediately following the telecast, Beard and Pickard attempted to assess any potential impact the *20/20* story might have on Sofamor Danek. This began in earnest on Saturday morning, the day after the telecast, when Pickard and a few other members of management met with Mike Cody, a Memphis attorney and former Tennessee Attorney General. Pickard had scheduled the meeting before the *20/20 program*—just in case, he said—but it ended up being more of a "chat" than a legal consultation. They all agreed that it was possible, even likely, that there would be no impact at all, so nothing specific came out of the meeting.

Although Beard was no longer involved in day-to-day operations at Sofamor Danek, he still maintained an office there, and several times during the next week he and Pickard discussed the matter at length. They reached no final conclusion, but each continued to believe there was no cause for alarm. Besides, at this point all they could do was wait and see. The whole thing might just blow over, at least as far as Sofamor Danek was concerned.

Pickard was further reassured when he spoke by phone with several independent financial analysts who had been following Sofamor Danek stock. These consultants had been developing reports so they could advise potential investors in the company, and most of thc feedback was good, along the lines of "Well, you guys probably don't have anything to worry about. You weren't mentioned." This added to what Pickard later acknowledged was a false sense of security on his part, and he began to enjoy the holidays.

Business was always slow at Sofamor-Danek in late December, what with Christmas and New Year's, and the year ground to a close without disruption. January also began quietly enough—at least until a deputy sheriff showed up at Pickard's home. The event would remain clear in his memory.

"It had to be well into the night. I woke up to somebody banging on the door, and I saw the blue lights. We lived in a little cove in Germantown. Anyway, I woke up and these lights were flashing, and I jumped up, put my pants on, and ran to the door. And there's this sheriff's guy, and he asked me if I was Ron Pickard. I said 'Yeah,' and he said, 'You're served!'"

Tennessee law requires every corporation doing business in the state to designate a registered agent for service of process, and Pickard was Sofamor Danek's registered agent. Still half asleep, he took the papers and read them. The company was being sued for injuries allegedly resulting from the use of the company's screws in spinal surgeries. The issue had clearly not blown over after all.

In fact, the summons that the officer handed Pickard turned out to be only the first of what would become a tsunami of lawsuits against Sofamor Danek, eventually numbering more than 6,000 before the litigation was finally concluded. And for the company, the stakes could hardly have been higher. No investor wants that level of uncertainty, and in the next 12 months alone the value of Sofamor Danek stock would slide from around $33 a share to one-third that level. Not that either Beard or Pickard needed that long to understand the seriousness of the situation they were facing: before the month was out, both knew they were in a war for the future of the company.

Assuming it had one.

CHAPTER THIRTEEN: A LAWSUIT NEARLY ENDS SPINE SURGERY

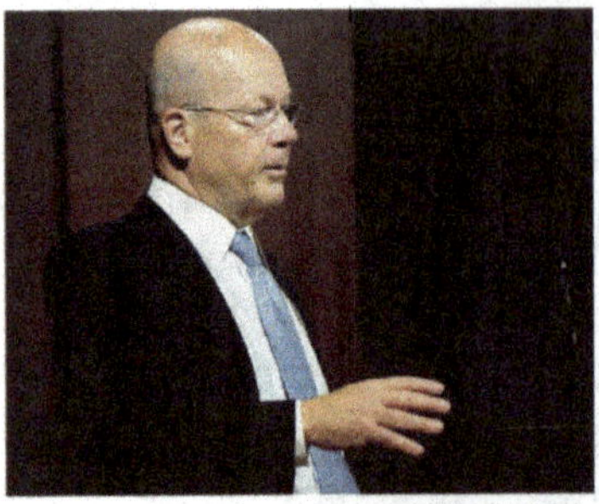

Steven Phillips, Lead Counsel, Sofamor Danek

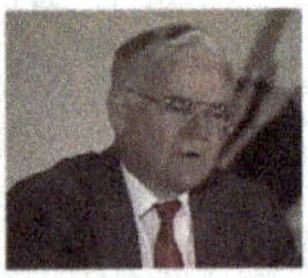

Judge Louis C. Bechtle

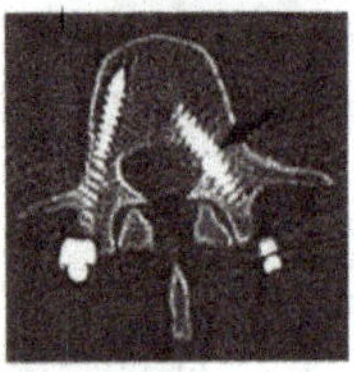

Broken Pedicle Screw
CT Scan.

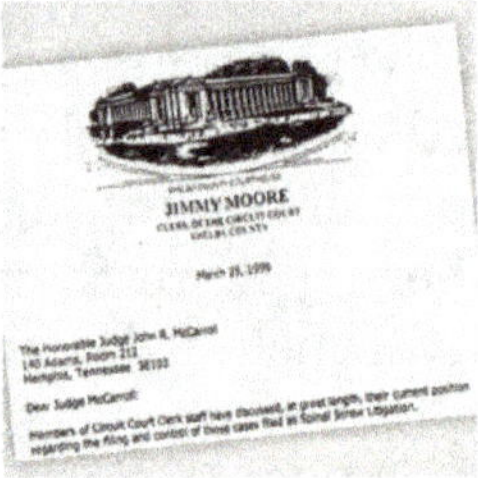

JIMMY MOORE
CLERK OF THE CIRCUIT COURT
SHELBY COUNTY

March 25, 199[illegible]

The Honorable Judge John R. McCarroll
140 Adams, Room 212
Memphis, Tennessee 38103

Dear Judge McCarroll:

Members of Circuit Court Clerk staff have discussed, at great length, their current position regarding the filing and control of those cases filed as Spinal Screw Litigation.

Letter from Shelby County Clerk's office to
Judge McCarroll.

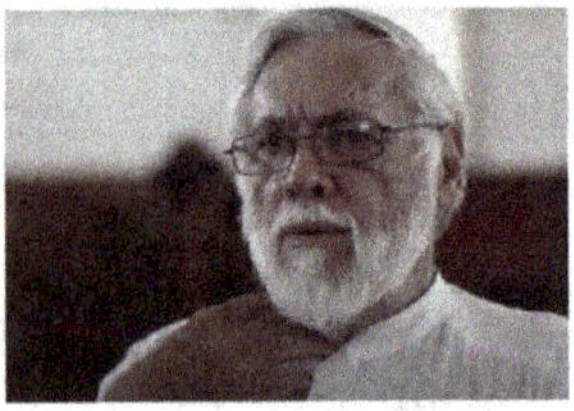

John Cummings, Lead Plaintiff Attorney,
Pedicle Screw Litigation.

In 1984 a woman named Maria Stern won $211,000 in compensatory damages and $1.5 million in punitive damages from a silicone breast manufacturer based in Memphis, Tennessee.

Ron Pickard, at the time, was president of the orthopaedic division of Richards Manufacturing.

That Memphis manufacturer of breast implants had been founded by a former Richards manufacturing's salesperson, Frank O. Wright 34 years earlier.

Wright Medical was at the time a division of Dow Corning Corporation. In addition to orthopedic products Wright made silicone breast implants. Frank O. Wright had died in February 1974 and his stepson, Robert (Bob) Rylee, ran the company.

The $1.5 million Stern ruling went largely unnoticed.

TV Commentators and Public Opinion vs Scientific Evidence

Eight years roll by.

A popular network tv program, *Face to Face with Connie Chung*, resurrected the Stern ruling and crafted a salacious story of greedy manufacturers, unethical surgeons and victimized patients. It was a sensational program which led Congress to hold hearings. More women filed lawsuits. Through their attorneys they claimed that leaking silicone breast implants caused cancer, autoimmune disorders and other illnesses—despite, it should be noted, literally no scientific evidence.

In July 1991 Brenda Toole won a $5.4 million settlement. In December, Mariann Hopkins received $7.3 million. Then things really got going.

CBS's powerhouse investigative program, *60 Minutes* aired the cases. Talk show host Phil Donahue interviewed women who were suing manufacturers. *Court TV* broadcast an entire silicone breast implant trial. The plaintiff's attorneys hired PR firms to keep the momentum going.

All over television breast implant manufacturers were painted as evil, greedy, and blind to patient suffering. Surgeons were incompetent at best, heartless at worst. The jury awards kept rising—reaching, by the end of 1992, $25 million ($20 million in punitive damages) per case. By the end of 1993, 12,359 breast implant cases were working their way through the courts.

In September 1993, the four breast implant manufacturers, desperate to end the onslaught negotiated a massive $4.75 billion settlement. But the new cases kept coming. The settlement deal collapsed. Dow Corning, Wright Medical's parent company filed for Chapter 11 bankruptcy. The remaining three manufacturers settled for $3.4 billion, the largest class action settlement up to that point.

Then scientific evidence began to emerge in the peer-review literature (not exactly mass media).

- *Plastic and Reconstructive Surgery* published a study that found no increase in the incidence of breast cancer in women who had received breast implants.
- The *New England Journal of Medicine* followed with a study that concluded that breast implants did not substantially increase a woman's risk for breast cancer.
- *New England Journal of Medicine* published a study by Mayo Clinic epidemiologists that found no increased risk of connective tissue disease in women with silicone gel breast implants.
- American College of Rheumatology issued a statement saying that the evidence is "compelling...silicone implants expose patients to no demonstrable risk for connective-tissue or rheumatic disease," and that "anecdotal

evidence should no longer be used to support this relationship in the courts or by the FDA."

- American Academy of Neurology reviewed existing silicone gel breast implant studies and concluded that there was no link between the implants and neurological disorders.
- *Journal of the National Cancer Institute* published a review of studies and concluded that breast implants did not cause breast cancer.
- After receiving input from a panel of impartial scientists, a federal judge from Oregon ruled that plaintiffs' evidence linking silicone implants to disease was scientifically invalid.
- An Alabama judge appointed a panel of scientific experts which, after two years and $800,000, concluded that breast implants did NOT cause disease.

Ultimately, the breast implant manufacturers won 80% of the cases. But it was too late for Dow Corning and its Memphis based medical products manufacturer, Wright Medical.

Bob Rylee, who'd been promoted to chairman of Dow Corning's medical products business had fought the good but losing fight as the company's principal spokesman trying to make the case that silicone breast implants were NOT causing disease.

Rylee had grown up on a farm in Denison, Texas, served in the U.S. Army and following a law degree from the University of Texas became a partner in a Corpus Christi law firm. During his years there, he was also a director of The Salvation Army, director of Preferred American Life Insurance Company and Casey & Glass Inc.

When Frank Wright died in 1974, Rylee pulled up stakes and relocated to Memphis to run the family business.

After Dow Corning declared bankruptcy, 64 year-old Rylee decided it was time to retire. He walked out of Wright Medical for the final time and with his wife Kay, moved to Sarasota, Florida, for a much calmer life.

Then Sofamor Danek's Ron Pickard called.

The Mass Tort Playbook

Breast implant manufacturers did win 80% of the cases. But the plaintiff's attorneys, who extracted billions of dollars and bankrupted a major corporation, won the war. Science, it turned out, wasn't the key to winning; prime time, network television was.

As the breast implant litigation settlements were being crafted (and cases wound down), the plaintiff's bar looked for another mass tort gold mine.

They found it in the very new field of spine surgery and a small Louisiana spine surgery lawsuit.

"If you're right, you're right. And you've got to stick by that."

Ron Pickard, Alan Olsen (Danek's founder) and Bob Rylee had known each other for years. "So, I called Bob", recalls Pickard, "and I said, 'Bob, I've got this problem'. I told him about the pedicle screw litigation, and I said, 'Would you be willing to come on board as a consultant in our Litigation Oversight Committee?' He agreed and he came on board."

Rylee told Pickard up front, "I can't tell you what to do, but I can tell you what not to do. The first thing is: if you're right, you're right. And you've got to stick by that."

The original pedicle screw case was filed by a Louisiana spine patient named Gosserand who'd been treated in October 1986 with an AcroMed "buttress clamp" and bone screws. Gosserand's attorney alleged that the spine fusion surgery had failed, and his client was owed damages. The jury agreed. On March 7, 1989, Gosserand was awarded $950,000—which was remitted on January 31, 1990, to $500.000.

Another Louisiana spine surgery lawsuit was filed by a St. Charles, Louisiana, patient, Dorothy Reeves, a former maid who, through her attorney, Darryl Tschim, said that after being treated with spinal fusion, which included using AcroMed's plates and pedicle screws to stabilize her spine, that she "hurt constantly" and was unable to work. "Several screws have broken," her attorney alleged. Reeves was awarded $475,000 in 1993 (later remitted to $410,000).

Literally two weeks after the *20/20* exposé, on New Year's Eve 1993, the plaintiff's attorneys filed the first putative class action against AcroMed.

Very quickly, that complaint was updated to include Sofamor Danek, and the sheriff turned up at Pickard's home late one night to serve the summons and complaint.

The second putative nationwide class action, representing over 100 class representatives as plaintiffs and targeting literally every supplier of bone screws in the world, was filed in the U.S. District Court for the Eastern District of Louisiana just weeks later.

The explicit threat to the ten relatively small spinal implant manufacturers was that these cases could balloon into more than 500,000 lawsuits which, if class actions, would create an overwhelming "asymmetrical risk" for each company.

The goal of the plaintiff attorneys, of course, was to win by forcing massive settlements regardless of the science or merits of any individual patient's claim.

"By the end of January or February we knew. It was an avalanche," remembers Pickard today. "The lawsuits kept coming in. The sheriff was showing up with these big plastic trays [of legal documents]. Out of my office you could look down and see them drive in."

Sofamor Danek needed a lawyer. What they were looking for was an unconflicted battlefield general. What they got was a born and bred Philadelphia lawyer who, they would learn, had a street fighter's instincts and grit—Pepper Hamilton's Stephen Phillips.

Don't Let the Other Side Get Between You and Your Customer

"It finally dawned on us what was happening with litigation about pedicle screws. We as a company made a couple decisions that, I think, were really instrumental in the outcome," recalls Pickard.

The first decision was to keep the legal fight bottled up and away from company operations and surgeon customers. Ironically, when the plaintiff attorneys decided to go after the surgeon societies (AAOS, NASS, SRS and others) and the surgeons themselves, it strengthened the ties between Sofamor Danek and the surgeon community. The goodwill that engendered, to this day, is one of the reasons Medtronic Spine is the #1 supplier in the industry.

"We formed a legal oversight committee separate from the management committee."

The committee consisted of L.D. Beard (Danek co-founder and board member), Ron Pickard (chairman and CEO), Alan Olsen (Danek co-founder), Bob Rylee (former chairman of Dow Corning Healthcare, attorney and chairman of the Legal Oversight Committee), Ken Kramer (attorney, Sherman & Sterling), Ed Basile (attorney, King & Spaulding) and Stephen Phillips (Sofamor Danek lead litigation attorney, member of the National Coordinating Council, EVP and General Counsel for Sofamor Danek).

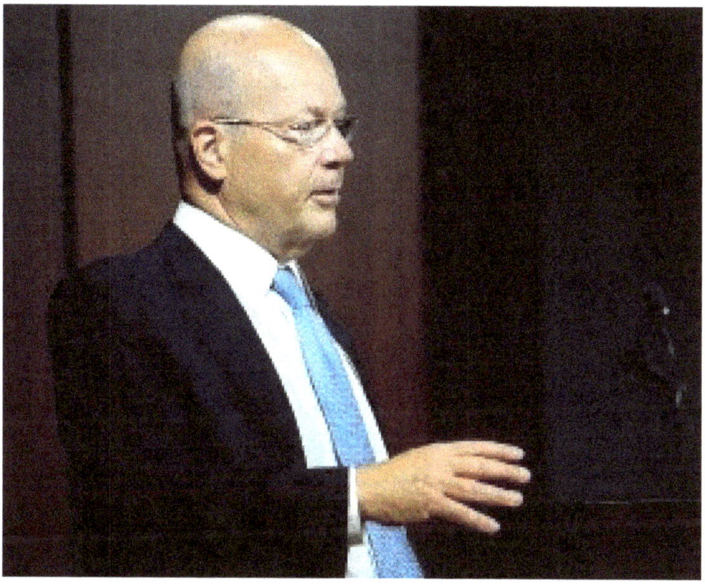

Stephen Phillips, Lead Counsel Sofamor Danek during Pedicle Screw Litigation

"We didn't talk about the litigation outside of the legal oversight committee. We were very strict on that fact," remembers Pickard.

When the plaintiff's started suing individual spine surgeons, Sofamor Danek's customers and their attorneys would call the company asking for help. Remembers Pickard, "Patient's doctors and their attorneys were calling us saying 'Look, can you help us with discovery information.'"

"Of course, our attorneys were saying 'No, no, you've got to shield yourself. You've got to let them run their litigation, you run ours.'"

But Bob Rylee stepped up and told Pickard and everyone else on the litigation committee "That's the biggest mistake we made at Dow Corning. We actually had a separation between us and the customer. Even though the science was not on plaintiff's side. They were able to divide us from our customer."

Pickard told his lawyers, "Yes, we're going to share information, yes, we're going to work with them. Figure out a way to do it. If there is a risk associated with that, we'll take that risk."

One surgeon in particular, Hansen Yuan, who was also at the time president of North American Spine Society, placed a late night call to Pickard personally. He told him, "I've run up all these bills at NASS. I've got more than $1 million of legal expense. NASS needs help."

The first thing Pickard told Dr. Yuan was, "Hansen, don't worry about it, I'll cover it." He hung up and thought to himself, "What in the devil did I just do?" He went the next morning to talk to his chief financial officer, Laurance Fairey, and told him what he'd done. Fairey reminded Pickard, "Don't you need board approval for that?" To which Pickard replied, "Probably, but it's done now."

Looking back, Pickard makes the point that while Sofamor Danek and NASS may have had different strategies, where it made sense, and when the strategies coincided, then "We were executing on the most important strategy of all, the one we had from Day One – *the customer is #1*."

'Burn the Ships'—There Is No Turning Back

The plaintiff's bar organized their cases around simple, powerful, and intuitively sensible arguments:

- The surgeries were unsuccessful. Patients, as the juries could plainly see, were experiencing terrible pain and too often permanently disabled.
- The pedicle screws were not FDA approved. An official FDA letter said that AcroMed's screws were "not substantially equivalent" to other spinal fixation devices. Further, said the FDA,

they posed “potential risks not exhibited by other spinal fixation systems,” including “screw failure.”

- Pedicle screws, said the FDA, required “premarket approval” before they could “be legally marketed” for spinal indications.
- Pedicle screw manufacturers, therefore, knowingly sold experimental, unapproved and therefore illegal implants which left patients permanently disabled.
- The companies, other surgeons, and the surgeon societies participated in this illegal activity by teaching surgeons to use these investigational, unapproved devices.

Plaintiffs' lawyers across the country competed with one another to gather clients, running newspaper advertisements, setting up toll-free telephone numbers to solicit patients. In a particularly outrageous move, the plaintiffs’ attorneys even tried to exhibit at NASS’ annual meeting as a subcontractor in another vendor’s booth!

Many years later, L.D. was asked if he had taken the allegations in the lawsuits personally. After all, plaintiffs were claiming that the company, his company, was putting profit ahead of patient health.

"I don’t guess I ever took it personally. I was always able to sort of compartmentalize myself and the company. What my personal feelings were versus what was good for business, what I owe the company, what I have to do for the company, what my position is in the company. Once we set everything in motion, I really just listened more than I did anything."

Setting everything in motion meant making some major organizational decisions within the company and driving this was the central issue: settle the lawsuits or engage in a fight with an uncertain outcome. And especially if there was to be a fight, who, should take the lead, who should have the responsibility seeing it through? Equally important, who would run the company in the meantime?

Pickard credits L.D. with putting the threshold issue in perspective: "Well, I listened to L.D. For example, L.D. said, 'You know, a company may be sold one day. Somebody may come along and buy it, but if you're thinking of selling the company, you can't build it at the same time. Your goal is to build it. And if someone comes along one day and thinks it's worth more than perhaps the shareholders do, whatever, that's fine. Your strategy is to build the company. If you build the company, build something of value, and somebody wants it, okay.' "

Building something of value, Pickard understood, should always be the goal. And to him it was clear that a legal settlement was a threat to that goal: "If we settle today, what are we going to be selling tomorrow? The same product. Or we close the doors. There's not another option. And that's the reason I couldn't understand AcroMed settling. This wasn't like Richards, where a bone screw was only part of their business."

L.D. thought the same even as he recognized the degree of uncertainty and that nobody could claim to know the outcome, including the lawyers.

"The lawyers didn't offer answers to any of the questions I had. In court defendant companies had always settled. So, nobody could provide the answers as to how winnable the cases were."

However, what was clear to L.D. and Pickard the enormous cost of fighting the lawsuits: "We're going to be spending money on attorneys and investigators and everything else, but we're growing so fast and we're earning so much, it's going to be cheaper dollars, because next year we're going to be making more money than we did this year as long as someone stays focused on business."

It might make the company less attractive to investors in the short run, but neither L.D. nor Pickard was focusing on the short run. They were determined not to surrender and not to settle. In L.D.'s mind it was the right decision because it was a business decision, and his view was reinforced as events unfolded:

"You have to remember two things. One is that in business, everything is a series of choices. So, we had no idea what it would take to settle the litigation, and I don't think the claimant's attorneys had any idea, either. We discussed settlement, but without a number. It's impossible to really determine what to do. We knew it would be up into the several hundred million dollar range, because they thought that they had good cases and that they could get something like the breast implants and that sort of thing."

"At that point we really didn't have any way of settling. Didn't know what it would take. We had cash, we had value, but we didn't have any means of knowing, and of course, once you approach with a settlement offer, you've set the stage for a lot of negotiating and a lot of, I'd say, misrepresentation about what the case is really worth. The idea gets to be if they want to settle, they must feel that they don't have much of a case. So, at that point I don't think we had a choice but to fight."

"And so, the choice became how to fight. And that was to be as aggressive as we could possibly be."

The Judicial Panel for Multidistrict Litigation consolidated all federal cases, including the putative class actions, and assigned them to Judge Louis C. Bechtle, Chief Judge Emeritus of the U.S. District Court for the Eastern District of Pennsylvania.

On February 22, 1995, Judge Bechtle denied class certification. The first piece of good news for the manufacturers.

For the defense, Sofamor Danek's lead counsel Stephen Phillips had to recruit a nation-wide network of lawyers covering the majority of Federal districts. Early on, he pulled them together at a meeting in Chicago which still sticks in Ron Pickard's mind.

"We called a meeting of all the lawyers from around the country. It was a lot of people. Lawyers and their associates. I had Alan Olsen come in. He actually did a saw-bones lab for the attorneys. After all, how can anyone represent us if they don't know what they are representing?"

"All these lawyers filled the auditorium at the Hilton in Chicago," remembers Pickard. "I was sitting in the back and Steve was running the meeting. For the first 30-45 minutes there were questions like 'if we enter into a settlement solution we go this route or that route.'"

"I finally raised my hand and said: 'Steve, can I say something?'

"'Sure', he said."

"So, I walked up front and said 'I don't want to be ugly, I don't want to be nasty, I don't want to be rude. But, if anyone has any questions or wants to discuss settlement, please leave now. Because that is not on the table."

"I don't know how you win if the first thing you talk about is how you lose. So, please, you won't hurt my feelings, if you want to talk about settlement, get the hell out of the room. Go on back home."

Then Pickard walked out of the room, went to the cafeteria, and ordered a cup of coffee.

"That," recalls Sofamor Danek's general counsel Phillips, "set the tone for the meeting and the entire litigation."

Jim Gallogly Takes Over as President and Chief Operating Officer

In 1993 L.D. was board chairman, and Pickard was president and CEO. L.D. was not interested in returning to run the company, let alone manage the legal struggle, and Pickard had his hands full with running the company. On the other hand, active leadership of the legal strategy was hardly something that could be outsourced. Ultimately, there was really only once even though it would mean some organizational changes. Changes which Pickard and the board made.

In early March of 1994, James Gallogly was brought on board as president and chief operating officer of the company, and Pickard remained as CEO. At the same time, L.D. stepped down as chair but remained on the board, and Pickard also was named the new chairman of the board. Gallogly's credentials spoke for themselves: he had once held the same position at Richards. Pickard was convinced that Gallogly was the right choice to handle daily operations:

"Jim could effectively run the company. He had the experience, the knowledge. A lot of people knew of Jim, had been associated with him, so he had an instant respect, if you will. He and I saw things the same way, so philosophically I had no hesitation about kind of stepping out of things."

"I stayed in the business mostly from the investment, the public market side of it. But from an operational point of view, I didn't have a lot of activity. I didn't get involved much. Jim ran it all."

Wall Street Analysts

Customers were not the only ones needing reassurance. Wall Street's financial analysts and institutional investors, mutual funds and pension funds were encountering real difficulty in completing a profile of the company, and Pickard saw the underlying problem:

"They can't do a financial model of this company without knowing a number, and they can't do their research. They can't make their predictions. They can't write their papers. And so they're just saying, 'Stay away. Stay away.'"

"So, I went to talk to L.D. I gave him my theory and he agreed with it. And I said, 'What if we come up with a number, and not say that that's what it's going to cost, but we're going to take a one-time charge.'"

"And when people say, 'Is that going to cover it?', we don't know—it's our best guess. And it's a paper transaction. We announced a fifty-million-dollar write-off. Within two weeks, our stock had doubled. That's the lesson I learned. Nothing fundamentally changed. We reported our primary results on a pro forma basis, and everybody said, 'Okay, there's that write-off now.'"

NASS, AAOS and Individual Surgeons Are Sued

"I don't remember exactly when we first were served with the pedicle screw litigation. Probably February of 1995," recalls Eric Muehlbauer, just six months in his new position as Director of the North American Spine Society. "We started to get boxes of lawsuits served on us. A box literally filled with 200 lawsuits. I had to sign for them. We ended up getting sued 522 times."

The plaintiff's theory was that since NASS had sold pedicle screw manufacturer's booth space, that the Society was party to commercializing unapproved spinal implants and therefore a fraud on the marketplace.

"It was shocking. I didn't expect to be, you know, under siege in my first six months on the job."

NASS'soffices were, at the time, still in the American Academy of Orthopaedic Surgeons (AAOS) building. NASS was one of AAOSs affiliate specialty societies and Muehlbauer had been hired by AAOS to transition NASS out of AAOS.

Rick Peterson, AAOS' attorney, who'd also been served, called Muehlbauer told him that NASS had to find a lawyer by one o'clock that same afternoon. All defendants to the litigation—the manufacturers and the societies—were holding a call in just a few hours.

By pure luck, Muehlbauer had met Shawn Collins, a litigator and CPA a few months earlier. Quick call and in in time for the afternoon meeting, NASS had their attorney.

"At first I was really just scrambling to understand what was going on and then look at what's our insurance coverage. Credit the Academy, they gave us great advice. At the peak of the litigation, we were getting bills of $125,000 a month."

Ultimately NASS' legal bills topped $2 million and all in, the litigation lasted about two years. "We ended up getting about $1.5 million of it back from our insurance carrier—but not without a fight, which is another story," remembers Muehlbauer.

During the litigation, the mass tort plaintiff attorneys tried to paint NASS' President, Dr. Hanson Yuan, as the lead surgeon "bad guy". NASS's counsel, Sean Collins saw it coming and, as Muehlbauer recalls, "went right at them", fighting tooth and nail, beating back even, for example, references to Dr. Yuan's ethnicity.

NASS counsel Collins and Director Muehlbauer never talked settlement. The Academy, however, briefly entertained the idea.

One meeting in particular stands out to Muehlbauer. "I remember there was a hearing that I had to attend in

Philadelphia in front of a three judge panel. At the court, before proceedings started, the AAOS attorney tried to introduce me to one of the other attorneys. I'm about to shake his hand and he is introduced to me as one of the plaintiff's attorneys. I didn't wanna shake his hand. I said, 'What are you doing?'"

Turns out, the AAOS attorney had been talking settlement—potentially at the expense of the other medical societies. AAOS' leadership eventually put a stop to those back channel conversations.

Muehlbauer credits certain surgeon leaders for helping him save NASS. "Hanson Yuan really stood up and was a leader, without a doubt."

"Jeff Saal, a physiatrist, he understood strategically how important it was for him to be kind of the mouthpiece for the surgeons. He didn't have a dog in the fight. He's not a surgeon. He never implanted a pedicle screw. But he was emphatic about medical education. About having exhibit booths. We can have clinical guidelines and things like that, and even talk to industry, but we are in control of our education, industry is not."

With these leaders, NASS never came close to throwing in the towel.

Finally, in 1996, the litigation ended for NASS. AcroMed negotiated a settlement with the plaintiffs' attorneys. "Sofamor Danek said they would never settle. We appreciated the fact that AcroMed wanted to extricate us from this," remembers Muehlbauer, "And we were released from those 522 lawsuits."

The AcroMed settlement caught the other defendants—Sofamor Danek, the other manufacturers and the surgeons who'd been sued—by surprise. It felt like a betrayal. Up until that point, AcroMed and the other parties had been cooperating in a joint defense.

Most galling, though, was the reality that those settlement dollars, roughly $100 million, would go to fuel the plaintiffs' continued mass tort extortion attempt.

How the Most Consequential Lawsuit in Medical History Was Won

While not the largest litigation in the history of medicine, the pedicle screw lawsuit is probably the most consequential. It which would eventually engulf all ten (at the time) manufacturers of spinal implants, every single surgeon society, the American Medical Association, thousands of individual spine surgeons and even the United States government. It would establish, once and for all, by way of a ruling from the United States Supreme Court, the primacy of physician decision making.

And yet, for all that, this landmark litigation started as a fairly typical malpractice case.

A St. Charles, Louisiana, patient, E.D. Gosserand, already suffering debilitating and disabling back pain, elected to have spinal fusion surgery in October 1986. The surgeon chose to implant a buttress clamp and bone screws, manufactured by Cleveland, Ohio based AcroMed Corporation as a method to stabilize Gosserand's spine, support fusion between the diseased vertebrae and relieve pain.

It was not a successful surgery. Gosserand not only reported continuing pain and loss of function, but, as the attorney claimed in the resulting lawsuit, one or more of the implanted screws had broken causing, he claimed, various complications. It was, in strictly legal terms, a fairly typical malpractice lawsuit.

The issues were straight forward: Did the surgeon act negligently or in any material way breach their professional duty? Were the implants defective?

Ultimately, the court ruled in favor of the patient, setting the award at $950,000, which was later reduced to $500,000.

Intended Use

During the discovery phase of that first trial, the plaintiffs' lawyer noticed that although the screws and plates used in the surgeries had been FDA cleared for marketing, their *"intended use"* and, therefore, *labeling* was limited to the "long bones" of the body (e.g., arms or legs). Not spine.

The FDA had even issued an official form letter stating that AcroMed's metal plates and bone screws were "not substantially equivalent" to other spinal fixation devices and posed "potential risks not exhibited by other spinal fixation systems," including "screw failure." AcroMed's pedicle screw, said the FDA, required premarket approval and were "investigational" devices.

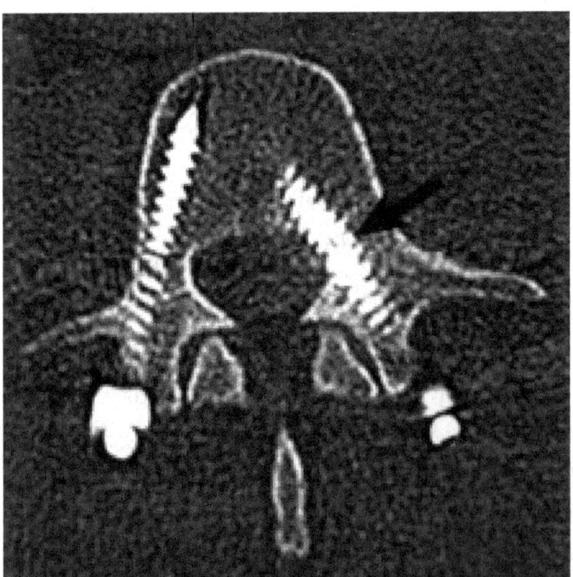

Broken Pedicle Screw CT Scan / Source: Research Gate

Spotting a novel theory of liability—namely, illegal marketing for an untended use—the Louisiana based lawyers, who had experience with mass tort litigation, were sure they'd stumbled across the next major class action case.

Stephen Phillips, Sofamor Danek's lead counsel at the time recalls, "That FDA letter provided the plaintiffs with a simple and alluring explanation of why the screws in a number of patients had broken. At the same time, it suggested that AcroMed's devices were being illegally marketed in the United States."

One lawsuit for every pedicle screw based spine surgery in the United States meant upwards of 500,000 cases—nearly 600 lawsuits *per* employee of the defending manufacturers.

Brandishing the "intended use" argument plaintiffs' attorneys began aggressively soliciting spine fusion cases from around the country. So aggressive were their tactics that, as we will see later, many of the lawsuits were filed were without the knowledge or even consent of their putative "clients."

The plaintiff attorney's goal was clear, turn a fairly typical malpractice case into mass class tort litigation. Had they succeeded in that effort and certified any of the putative classes, they would have created an overwhelming, asymmetrical advantage of more than half million pedicle screw lawsuits.

As Phillips remembers, "The sheer magnitude of the financial risk facing all of the companies would have been overwhelming. Creating such "asymmetrical" risk—which is precisely the objective of the lawyers asserting such claims—that the industry would have been forced to agree to a "global" settlement regardless of the merits of any individual claim."

The First Major Plaintiff Loss: Class Certification Denied

Within two weeks of the *20/20* broadcast, the first of eight putative class actions were filed. The federal cases were consolidated in 1994 assigned to 72-year-old U.S. District Judge Louis C. Bechtle in Philadelphia. Judge Bechtle was nationally recognized for his ability to organize, drive, even bully, complex mass tort cases to resolution.

In order to qualify litigation as a "class" attorneys have to prove that there exists a natural commonality among the plaintiffs. Each claim, essentially, has to assert the identical theory of liability. For example, if the lawsuit is about buying stocks, then, while the amount of an individual investment might vary, the individual investor liability question can be identical. Identical plaintiff theories of liability are pre-requisite for class certification.

The identical liability test failed before Judge Bechtle—for three reasons. First, no two patient pathologies or circumstances are exactly alike. Second, there were widespread differences between individual surgeon diagnosis and treatment plans—even for the same pathology, again reflecting the unique combinations of patient and surgeon. Finally, as Phillips explained, "Every one of these manufacturers who makes these orthopedic bone screws had a different regulatory history. They were simply not identical."

There was no alternative for Judge Bechtle and on February 22, 1995, he denied the plaintiff's motion for class certification.

With the possibility of a class action gone, a cascade of individual lawsuits against the ten manufacturers of bone screws, plates and rods rolled in. Cases were filed in both federal and state courts.

Now the lawyers representing patients had to argue theories of liability for each patient's case individually—which, as it would turn out, made facts, Sofamor Danek's asymmetrical advantage, the determinant of the bone screw litigation outcomes.

Judge Louis C. Bechtle Takes Charge

As L. Stuart Ditzen wrote in his excellent August 2000 article in the *Philadelphia Inquirer Magazine*, "[Judge Bechtle] has wrestled several mass cases to resolution over the years. One of Bechtle's techniques is to drive the litigation toward trial on a brutally strict timetable. That pressure can be the catalyst that brings on a settlement."

Stephen Phillips remembers; "Judge Bechtel ordered for discovery purposes that we complete over 1,200 depositions in four months! At one point we had 42 law firms working under my direction as the National Coordinating Counsel. These 42 law firms were doing 2, 3, 4 depositions a day for four months straight."

"Keeping track of every single deposition, which attorneys were going where and getting witnesses and others prepared and producing the documents...was, no pun intended...back breaking. Which was, actually, Bechtle's objective."

Phillips, who'd appeared before Bechtle in other mass tort cases, recognized the tactic immediately. "Bechtle's tactic was to make unreasonable demands as a way of facilitating early collapse by the defendants and forcing a settlement."

Phillips and his army of attorneys did it. Four months later, 1,200 depositions—and ALL the critical information that they brought to the defense lawyers—were completed, catalogued, analyzed and ready.

"I don't think there are many people who would have gotten through that gauntlet in that interval of time," says Phillips today.

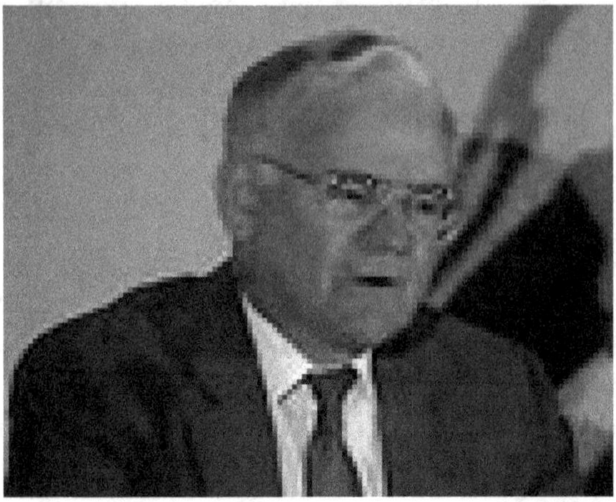

Judge Louis C. Bechtle / Source: C-Span

Attacking the "Defective Device" Claim

During this period, a group of Sofamor Danek shareholders also filed suit against their own company, basically claiming that company management had intentionally and routinely withheld or downplayed the risks of its own activities and the risks of the litigation itself, which in turn had resulted in financial losses to those shareholders. Sofamor Danek denied this and cited its own public statements that, it said, gave ample notice of the various risks. Courts of law would ultimately decide the issues.

But neither Ron Pickard nor L.D. Beard could have anticipated the protracted legal siege that took place during the months, and, as it would turn out, the years following the *20/20* telecast. And their lack of genuine worry was understandable. As Pickard later recalled, "We weren't mentioned [in the segment]. It was AcroMed. We had only one lawsuit in the history of the company, and it was over a broken instrument. It didn't have anything to do with implants."

By 1995, the plaintiffs had filed 3,238 cases against Sofamor Danek alone—nearly 2,000 at the state level (more than 1,700 in Tennessee and more than 200 in Oklahoma). Bechtle's order to depose 1,200 litigating patients over four months had given Phillips and his team a treasure trove of information about the plaintiff's clients and their cases.

Remembers Phillips, "We obtained tremendous amount of information. We learned about the plaintiff's clients and each case. We analyzed the data. We looked at all the medical records of the people in the cases and we found out, well, wait a minute, only 11% of these plaintiffs have broken devices."

In other words, 89% of the patients did not have broken screws—which was the basis for the defective device theory of liability. Furthermore, Sofamor Danek's medical consultants were certain that broken screws in most patients were *asymptomatic.*

According to Sofamor Danek's experts, pain, when it did manifest, was generated from movement between the vertebrae—which were intended to fuse and, therefore, not move.

In more than two-thirds of the cases, the devices, the bone screws, performed as expected. "Why, we wondered, are we in a lawsuit with an army of patients who got the result that they expected?" recalls Phillips.

Even with a broken screw, a significant number of patients nonetheless went on to experience fusion. Furthermore, the medical records of 26% of Sofamor Danek's plaintiffs showed that their devices had loosened, but most of them also eventually obtained fusion. The devices in the remaining 63% of its plaintiffs experienced no failures or malfunctions and in most of these cases the plaintiff went on to obtain fusion.

Phillips and his team countered the defective device argument with the plaintiffs' own data that Sofamor Danek's bone screws were not responsible for the harm plaintiffs were claiming.

To put a final nail in the argument, Phillips and his team of 42 attorneys argued successfully that these lawsuits were an inappropriate attempt to convert manufacturers into guarantors of successful surgical outcomes.

Phantom Cases

In January 1998, surprisingly, 600 of the approximately 1,700 plaintiffs who'd filed lawsuits in Shelby County Circuit Court in Memphis asked Judge John R. McCarroll, Jr. to dismiss their cases. As Ditzen wrote in his superb August 2000 *Philadelphia Inquirer* article, "Lawyers for Sofamor Danek decided to find out why: Pepper Hamilton's [the lead law firm representing Sofamor Danek and Stephen Phillips' firm] investigators interviewed and took written statements from 60 [of the patients who'd abandoned their cases]."

"Most of the 60 said they had been prompted by newspaper ads to call lawyers. Twenty-eight said they didn't know their names had been used in the lawsuits. Several of those individuals were interviewed for this story and confirmed that they did not know they were named as plaintiffs."

Here are three examples from Ditzen's article:

- "Phyllis Gaske of Sunnyvale, California, said she and her husband had seen a newspaper ad and called to get more information. "We never spoke with an attorney on the phone or in person," Gaske said, "They pursued us...We wrote a letter back informing them we were not interested...We have never sued anyone...We didn't intend to pursue a lawsuit because I was doing well, and it would have seemed fraudulent. We wouldn't do that."
- "I never had a face-to-face meeting with any attorneys," said Mark K. Halverson of Coon Rapids, Minnesota, whose chronic back pain

had led to four surgeries. "There was no difference between when the screws were in and when they were out, no difference whatsoever. So, the screws weren't the problem. The screws saved me from being in a body cast for six months...I was surprised to learn I had been part of a lawsuits..."

- "Deborah Scheers of McDonald, Pennsylvania, said she responded to a newspaper ad and filled out some papers mailed to her. "I also included a statement saying that I didn't want to be part of a lawsuit. I told them the screws worked for me and I was very happy with them. They gave me my life back..."

Then, in the Federal court in Philadelphia two of the plaintiffs' lawyers, Roy E. Amedee, Jr. and Andrea S. Lestelle, submitted hundreds of plaintiff questionnaires that contained false or obviously omitted information. Again, as Ditzen wrote in his *Philadelphia Inquirer* magazine article, "For example, one question was, 'Do you smoke?' The answer entered on numerous questionnaires was 'no', though many claimants, evidence would show, the answer should have been 'yes'"

Judge Bechtle imposed a $126,500 fine and sanctioned both Amedee and Lestelle saying, "I think it's unprofessional and I think it could violate the professional code of ethics."

Separating FDA Myth From FDA Reality

The plaintiffs' lawyers wanted to label the cases; "Unapproved Use Litigation"—which played on a widespread public misconception that the FDA approved the ways in which medical products are used. The FDA does not do that.

The FDA did not go to medical school, does not diagnose, or treat patients, does not engage in the practice of medicine.

Eventually, Bechtle agreed to name the lawsuits "Bone Screw Litigation."

"The argument that was being made was first that the FDA had not approved—keyword '*approved*'—orthopedic bone screws for use in the spine," recalls Phillips, "The way that sentence was structured, we knew, was false and very misleading."

"The FDA does not approve the *use* of medical devices. The FDA is only authorized to and has statutory authority to regulate the *marketing* and the *labeling* of devices, not how they are used."

Under the plaintiffs' attorney's malpractice theory, each spine surgeon had an obligation to inform their patients that they planned to make an off-label use of a device. Absent that explanation, the plaintiffs' attorneys argued, the surgery lacked informed consent. It was battery.

The plaintiffs' attorneys, therefore, pushed to expand informed consent to include FDA labeling issues as well as medical risks.

That, in turn, put manufacturers—potentially—at odds with their customers: spine surgeons.

FDA marketing clearances or approvals are negotiated between manufacturers and the FDA. Surgeons are not involved. Potentially, then, surgeons could be liable for something they weren't part of nor had control over.

To take that issue off the table, Ron Pickard, Sofamor Danek's CEO, decided to support any spine surgeons who'd been sued.

Defending Spine Surgeon's Ability to Practice Medicine

"Under Pickard's direction, Sofamor Danek collected every authoritative legal source concerning 'off-label' use, no matter how far afield," recalls Phillips, "and compiled these into legal arguments in support of spine surgeon's ability to practice medicine and defeat the false claims of lack of proper informed consent."

Phillips advanced these defenses of spine surgeons' rights in *amicus curiae* briefs in Ohio and California and in a partial summary judgment motion filed on behalf of surgeons in the federal Multi-District Litigation (MDL) proceedings before Judge Bechtle. Phillips then converted the extensive off-label use research generated by the litigation into an authoritative law review article, the first ever on the subject (Beck & Azari, "FDA Off-Label Use, and Informed Consent: Debunking Myths and Misconceptions." 53 Food & Drug L. J. 71 (1998) (Tab 300)).

According to Phillips, "Sofamor Danek's effort to help surgeons defeat the plaintiffs' unprecedented regulatory informed consent claims with *amicus curiae* briefs on critical issues, while unusual, was essential to the successful defense of surgeons and device manufacturers alike."

"Starting with the regulatory informed consent issue and expanding into preemption and class action tolling of the statute of limitations issues, Sofamor Danek made its attorneys available, at considerable expense, to advocacy organizations interested in appearing as *amicus* in selected cases."

"Among the *amici* Sofamor Danek assisted in this fashion were the American Medical Association (and several state affiliates), the American Hospital Association, the Medical Device Manufacturers

Association, the Product Liability Advisory Council, and in one case, the American Civil Liberties Union."

The strategy worked extremely well.

The Ohio Court of Appeals cited one of Sofamor Danek's earliest *amicus* briefs when they approved the first appellate decision rejecting regulatory informed consent.

That opinion, then, led to a summary judgment against the same theory in the federal MDL proceedings and was soon followed by similar decisions in California, Minnesota, Florida, Wisconsin, North Carolina, Tennessee, Pennsylvania, and New Jersey. The only appellate court that ever adopted plaintiffs' regulatory informed consent theory was subsequently reversed.

Goofball "Experts"

Having made the claim that bone screws caused their clients' injuries, pain and suffering, the attorneys were, naturally, required to present evidence. They needed experts.

The plaintiffs' lawyers were able to dredge up a small platoon of experts who would support their claims: Dr. Merrill Reuter, Dr. Lance Yarus, Dr. William Mitchell, Dr. Robert Pennell, Dr. Trobiani, Dr. Richard Bennett, and Dr. Antonio Aldrete.

Of them all, the most catastrophic—for the plaintiffs' attorneys—was Dr. Merrill Reuter, an orthopedic surgeon from West Palm Beach, Florida, who'd been recruited by a Sherman, Texas based former dermatologist, John S. Ferguson.

Ferguson, whose medical license was revoked following his conviction for illegal drug prescribing, served jail time in the 1980s and thereafter made a living finding medical experts for lawyers.

About 20 of the plaintiffs' attorneys engaged Ferguson to recruit medical experts. He found Merrill W. Reuter.

For $200 per case, Ferguson agreed to provide Reuter's expert medical opinions for individual plaintiffs the lawyers represented.

As Ditzen described in his 2000 *Philadelphia Inquirer* article: "He [Reuter] cranked out about 550 of them [reports]. He did not examine the surgery patients. He did not speak with them. He did not talk to their doctors. He [Reuter] testified in depositions that he formed his opinions from medical records sent to him by Ferguson."

A woman working in Reuter's office, Cynthia Adams, discovered tape recordings of John Ferguson dictating bone screw reports to Reuter. Adams, who had been involved with correspondence between Dr. Reuter and John Ferguson, called Ferguson to ask about the tapes. In her subsequent court deposition, she testified that Ferguson said to her: "Oh, my Lord, destroy those MF'ing tapes. If anyone gets ahold of those tapes, that's going to be the end of this..."

When Judge Bechtle found out, he barred all 550 of Dr. Reuter's opinions from being introduced as evidence in the bone screw litigation.

"The loss of Dr. Reuter as a witness was a significant blow to plaintiffs and severely impaired their ability to raise the triable issues needed to oppose our motions for summary judgment," remembers Phillips.

Ending 1,200 Tennessee Lawsuits With a Single Letter

The Federal cases in Judge Bechtle's court in Philadelphia were cranking forward in their own bureaucratic eco-system, but down in Memphis, in Judge John R. McCarroll's court, a different strategy was emerging—one that would end 1,200 bone screw lawsuits with a single, shocking, out-of-left-field letter.

As it happened, roughly 1,200 individual cases had been filed in the Shelby County Clerk's office as four separate 'class-action' lawsuits—which meant that the plaintiffs paid only four filing fees to cover approximately 1,200 cases.

Sofamor Danek's lead attorney, Stephen Phillips, was reluctant to call out his counterpart for gaming the system. "Judge John McCarroll was a southern gentleman of the first order," remembers Phillips. "And he was of the personal opinion that if you were a lawyer appearing before him, he would *per se* assume you are a person of integrity."

Phillips had earlier challenged the integrity of one of the plaintiff's attorneys and Judge McCarroll made his displeasure known.

So, Phillips found himself in an awkward position of knowing that the plaintiff's attorneys had misfiled approximately 1,200 cases—but felt he could not raise the issue in McCarroll's court.

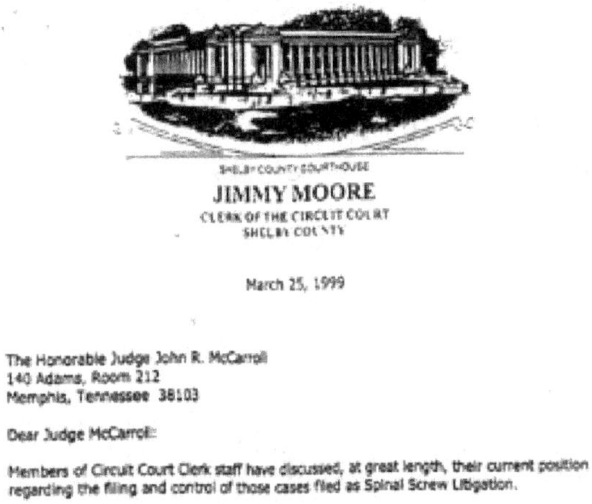

SHELBY COUNTY COURTHOUSE

JIMMY MOORE

CLERK OF THE CIRCUIT COURT
SHELBY COUNTY

March 25, 1999

The Honorable Judge John R. McCarroll
140 Adams, Room 212
Memphis, Tennessee 38103

Dear Judge McCarroll:

Members of Circuit Court Clerk staff have discussed, at great length, their current position regarding the filing and control of those cases filed as Spinal Screw Litigation.

Letter from Shelby County Clerk's office to Judge McCarroll
Courtesy of Steven Phillips

But he had remembered that the county clerk's staff were struggling with the sheer magnitude of all these cases, and it occurred to him that they might well NOT be aware of the misfiling, intentional or not.

Phillips called his Memphis co-counsel, Sam Blair, a long-time Memphis attorney (a Baker Donelson partner) who knew his way around the Shelby County Court. He asked Blair to have what amounted to an off-the-record 'chat' with the head of the County Clerk's office, Jimmy Moore, which Blair did.

Moore, in turn, investigated the "putative" class-certified bone screw cases and, sure enough, found they'd been misfiled. Furthermore, he confirmed that Shelby had been shorted hundreds of thousands of dollars in unpaid filing fees.

His response was an instant classic.

Under the official imprimatur of the Clerk of Circuit Court, Shelby County, Tennessee, Jimmy Moore and five senior members of his staff, including the Chief Accounting Officer, Administrator, two Deputy Administrators and Manager of the Cost Department, wrote a letter to Judge McCarroll on March 25, 1999, saying:

> "The Spinal Screw Litigation has not been established as a class-action lawsuit. Therefore, each case should be filed separately and filing fees collected for each file opened."
>
> "The current cases should be dismissed with costs assessed. All court costs incurred up to the filing of this dismissal order would be included in this order and would be assessed against one or more of the parties. When this order is entered, the Circuit Court Clerk would create a complete bill of costs. These costs would be due and payable to the Clerk of Circuit Court within 30-days of the date of this order."

As Phillips remembers today, "Jimmy Moore's letter was like the declaration of independence. He was saying, 'Dear judge, it's come to our attention that these cases are all misfiled. Here's what you gotta do. You gotta dismiss 'em all. Then let them refile one by one.' It was really cool."

Judge McCarroll issued an order shortly after receiving Moore's letter, dismissing all of the cases without prejudice with permission to be refiled individually, plaintiff by plaintiff...and pay the required filing fees.

None were ever refiled. 1,200 cases disappeared.

Game, Set, Match

From the start, the plaintiffs' lawyers said that they would not settle for any amount less than a billion dollars. One of the lead plaintiff's attorneys, John Cummings, literally demanded from Sofamor Danek "all the money" the company could possibly raise in return for which he would allow SDG "to remain in business."

When Judge Bechtle dealt the plaintiffs their first major defeat by denying class certification in February 1995, the settlement amount changed. In the summer of 1996, the plaintiffs' lawyers offered $150 million to both AcroMed and Sofamor Danek ($300 million total) to settle. Sofamor Danek, under Ron Pickard's leadership, flatly rejected the offer. AcroMed, who was buckling under the financial strain of the litigation, in December 1996, agreed to settle for $100 million.

The plaintiffs, thinking that they had the advantage, raised their settlement demand to Pickard and his company to $250 million. That was also rejected.

In 1997, lead plaintiff attorney, John Cummings proposed that Sofamor Danek settle all of its cases by issuing $225 million of convertible debentures. It was, given the gains Phillips and his litigation team were achieving in court, a ludicrous demand and flatly rejected.

In the summer of 1997, Judge Bechtle decided to use the power of the bench to drive the parties to a settlement and asked Phillips, "How much would Sofamor Danek be willing to pay to settle these cases?"

Sofamor Danek's litigation team calculated, essentially, the nuisance value of the outstanding claims and gave Judge Bechtle a dramatically reduced settlement number.

The plaintiffs responded by saying that the verdict value of all the outstanding federal cases was more than $2.4 billion. On March 20, 1998, Pickard, through Phillips, gave the Plaintiff's 10 days to accept the company's offer. The plaintiffs missed the deadline.

Court decisions kept mounting in Sofamor Danek's favor, week after week. Of the more than 3,700 bone screw cases filed in state and federal courts around the United States, only 176 made it to a judicial conclusion and of those, only one went against Sofamor Danek. That occurred in state court in Houston, Texas, where the plaintiff won a verdict of $413.000—which was affirmed on appeal. In one other case, Sofamor Danek lost, but that was later reversed on appeal.

Every other case was either withdrawn or dismissed.

Summary judgement decisions in favor of Sofamor Danek were rendered by 91 different judges, 73 in federal court (143 cases), 18 in state court (32 cases) and more than 50 appeals were initiated of which 14 were affirmed and 36 were pending at the time the plaintiffs capitulated.

Of the 3,200 individual claims that were filed against SDG, more than 70% were voluntarily dismissed.

The plaintiffs' lawyers basically surrendered. They agreed to end virtually all of the federal and related individual cases for a small fraction of the cost of litigating any of them.

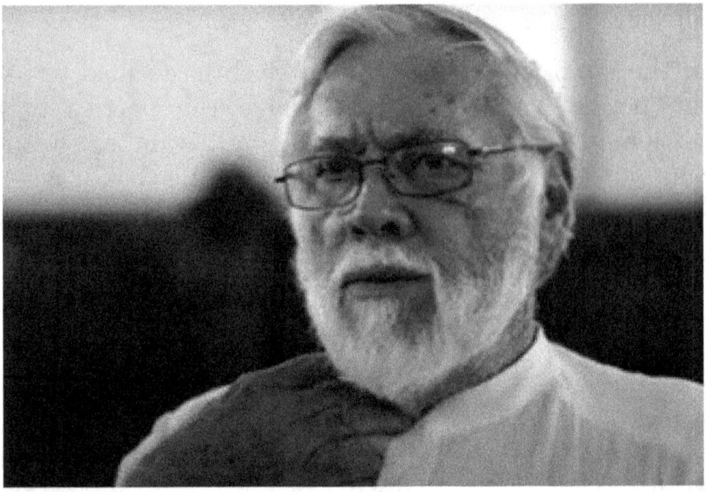

John Cummings, Lead Plaintiff Attorney
Pedicle Screw Litigation / Source: YouTube

The Toll

The fight lasted seven years, and L.D. later estimated the legal fees at about $125 million, but he did not doubt that it was worth it. After some initial setbacks, it was undeniable that the company was growing and continually becoming stronger. And he gave full credit to Pickard for this. But it must be noted that Pickard in turn gave credit to his mentor.

Both men would later admit to doubts, especially at the beginning. For Pickard in particular, the "war" was an almost constant drain, and there were times that he thought, "Maybe the best thing for me to do is just see if somebody else can't come in and do this better. You know, you do get burned out."

At the time, the problems seemed to be unending: "There was so much working against you. The system is working against you. The government is working against you. You don't fight that. You try to work your way through it. You take one step back and get knocked back three—or one step forward and get knocked back three. You know, we'd win a little skirmish here and win a little battle over here, and then all of a sudden some judge would rule some cockamamie thing in discovery that would drive you crazy."

And on one occasion his frustration would land him in court.

It occurred when he learned that AcroMed had settled. He couldn't believe it when Phillips told him. Pickard had met with AcroMed only two days earlier, and there had been no talk of settlement. He was furious, not so much at AcroMed as at the situation that had led them to its decision to settle, and his anger showed in a letter he sent out through the FAX database.

"I used the word 'extortion,' and the plaintiffs' attorneys took exception to that and went to Judge Bechtol in Philadelphia and said that I was calling them extortionists and inferring that the court was extorting people."

"And [the judge] got all worked up and ordered me to come to his courtroom. He had never addressed me directly. I just had to be there. He addressed Steve, our counsel on record, and he began to chew Steve out, and he said he would not tolerate this company calling him and his court contributing to extortion. And he goes on and on and on, and we're not going to put up with that, it's not helpful to the process, and he didn't want to hear about it anymore. Kind of implied he'd hold us in contempt, but Steve said he thought he'd never do that."

And what did Pickard do?

"So, we went back the next day, and I wrote another letter, and I used the same word. Extortion."

The Long-term Effect of the Pedicle Screw Litigation

There were, arguably, six significant long-term effects of the pedicle screw litigation:

1. Once and for all, the legal right of physicians to use medical devices and prescription drugs off-label without fear of exposure to liability was affirmed. In 1997, three years before the cases were resolved (!), under CEO Ron Pickard's leadership, Sofamor Danek lobbied Congress to amend the FDCA to state explicitly that nothing in the Act gave the FDA authority to regulate the practice of medicine by physicians. In 2001, the United States Supreme Court relied upon both this statute and the law review article written by Sofamor Danek's legal counsel to put to rest any doubt regarding the propriety of off-label use:

   > "'[O]ff-label' usage of medical devices (use of a device for some other purpose than that for which it has been approved by the FDA) is an accepted and necessary corollary of the FDA's mission to regulate in this area without directly interfering with the practice of medicine. [citing article]. Indeed, a recent amendment to the FDCA expressly states in part that "[n]othing in this chapter shall be construed to limit or interfere with the authority of a health care practitioner to prescribe or administer any legally marketed device to a patient for any condition or disease within a legitimate health care practitioner-patient relationship."

2. Sofamor Danek's unflinching support of surgeons and their professional societies cemented Sofamor Danek (later Medtronic Spine's) reputation as the most trusted

supplier in the spine and neuro sectors of medicine.

3. Competition from much larger, wealthier orthopaedic suppliers like DePuy, Stryker, Zimmer or Biomet was effectively delayed during the 4-years of this litigation.
4. Ron Pickard's decision to isolate the litigation from day-to-day operations of Sofamor Danek preserved customer relations and allowed the company to continue to innovatively move the practice of spine surgery forward—notably to develop the first surgical navigation system (Stealth Station) and to develop the first practical bone morphogenic protein, BMP2.
5. Ron Pickard's steadfast commitment to a simple rule—"If you're right, you're right and stick by that"—gave focus, backbone and inspiration to his team of lawyers and they, in turn, literally saved the practice of spine surgery.
6. Many of the frontline executives at Sofamor Danek, individual spine surgeons and executives of the surgeon societies remember this experience with enduring anger. They were slandered and liabled. At one point, when his patience finally broke, CEO Pickard characterized the entire plaintiff's activities as extortion—which it clearly was.

Medtronic Buys Sofamor Danek for $3.7 Billion

Medtronic had started out in 1949 as a medical equipment repair firm, but by the 1960s it had become a major player in the biomedical market, primarily through its battery-operated pacemaker. Over time, it brought onto market new products and acquired other companies, and in 1989 its total sales were above $1 billion. It was looking to expand into other implant markets by purchasing an orthopedic manufacturer. And not just any orthopedic manufacturer.

There were at least two reasons for Medtronic's interest. First, with the bone screw litigation winding down, Sofamor Danek was probably in its strongest position ever. In fact, its sales and income growth were remarkable. Second, Medtronic wanted to expand into the neurology business, and spinal implants seemed a logical platform on which to build. It also probably did not hurt that Sofamor Danek had withstood a litigation storm that would have swamped a less ably lead company.

The situation was far different from what it had been when Medtronic had first taken a look at Sofamor Danek. Ten years earlier Medtronic's leadership had met with L.D. to explore options, but it had not progressed beyond the talking stage. As L.D. later phrased it, "I think we were just a little too small for them at that time, and they didn't know what to do with it."

Things were now much changed, however, and one day Pickard's secretary called L.D. to ask if she could give someone his telephone number. Someone from Medtronic. L.D. told her it was okay, and soon after that the president of Medtronic's neurosurgery division called him, saying that he said he had been asked by Bill George, Medtronic's CEO, if he knew Ron Pickard. He had said no, but that he did know L.D. Beard, who could arrange a meeting. L.D. told him how to get in touch with Pickard.

The meeting took place in New York, but it was low-key. Pickard would later recall that the conversation was very general in nature:

"We had actually a cup of coffee in their suite. And they

chatted a little bit about the company and how they, you know, we were kind of on the periphery of the spine and neurosurgery business over here. Anyway, nothing really came of it."

Not at the time, at least, but that was not the end of it. George called Pickard again to ask if Pickard would be able to come to Minneapolis, a kind of "follow-up" to their New York meeting. Pickard agreed, and at this second meeting George told Pickard what he wanted: namely, Sofamor Danek. George also wanted Pickard's views on how the rest of Sofamor Danek's management, particularly L.D., would respond to the idea. Pickard thought he knew but was noncommittal: "I think L.D. is a shareholder, and he'll do what's right for the shareholders."

Pickard was more direct when he met with L.D. after his return from Minneapolis. He wanted L.D. to take the lead on any negotiations, partly because Pickard had acquired various stock options over the years, and he felt it would be inappropriate for him to be involved in negotiations. L.D. met with senior Medtronic managers in the summer of 1998. L.D. went alone.

Because the negotiations had to remain secret, L.D. used an assumed name, and both sides immediately agreed on one goal: any merger must not negatively impact shareholders in either company.

As always, L.D. had done the math in advance:

'I had already looked at their numbers and everything, and I said, 'Well, I know what the price should be.' And it was about forty or fifty dollars more than we were selling for at the time, I think, something like that. We were in the seventy-five to eighty range, and it looked like [the purchase price] was going to be somewhere in the range of a hundred and twenty dollars. And I just named off that number."

And L.D. had other one other condition. He was determined that Sofamor Danek would not end up on an auction block. "If you are all interested, don't send a corporate jet loaded with accountants down to swarm all over the place. We both have the same accounting firm, so it will be easy to do your due diligence. I want it done quickly and quietly, and I don't want the company to be in play."

Both sides knew a good deal, and the following January the deal was finalized. L.D. had celebrated his 66th birthday a month earlier, and now he could leave on his own terms. And he never doubted that the merger was a good idea:

"I thought the timing was right. We had an opportunity to sell to a good company, a highly regarded company, and a company we were somewhat familiar with from past dealings, and we were at the point ourselves where we would need to become probably more aggressive in our management staff."

It was a task that L.D. was more than willing to leave to others. It had been an exhausting five years not only for him and Pickard, but for so many Sofamor Danek board members and executives.

As for Pickard, he had no plans to leave Sofamor Danek, but the leadership at Medtronic changed, and the unwritten understandings between him and George did not continue after George left:

"Bill [George] and I had a lot of discussion about, you know, we don't really want to change Sofamor Danek. 'Clearly, you're not going to be a public-traded company. You're not going to have your own board of directors. But, you know, we really don't want to impede your growth. There are certain corporate rules and guidelines you've got to fall into, but they're more financial than anything else.'"

"But when Bill left, there was no memory of those discussions. My last trip to Medtronic was at the request of the new CEO who had just recently succeeded Bill George."

We had dinner in his club that was closed that night, but he had arranged for a dinner with just the two of us in the club restaurant. Over dinner I learned that he had never supported Medtronic's purchase of Sofamor Danek. But, he said, the deal was done. Going forward, he told me, I was expected to fall in line with the Medtronic program. Period. No discussion."

"I did not respond or comment to him. I went back to Memphis and began to clear out my office."

"Medtronic engaged in a pretty aggressive onslaught at Sofamor Danek that first year.'

Years later, Pickard was philosophical about the unwelcome changes: "I'd been around long enough to know that you may not think you're exhibiting a negative attitude, but everyone around you will. And so I felt the best thing for me to do before that happened is to get out. I could get out, and my life could go on."

Pickard left Medtronic Spine (formerly Sofamor Danek) before the year was out.

CHAPTER FOURTEEN: THE GOLDEN AGE FOR ORTHOPAEDICS AND SPINE

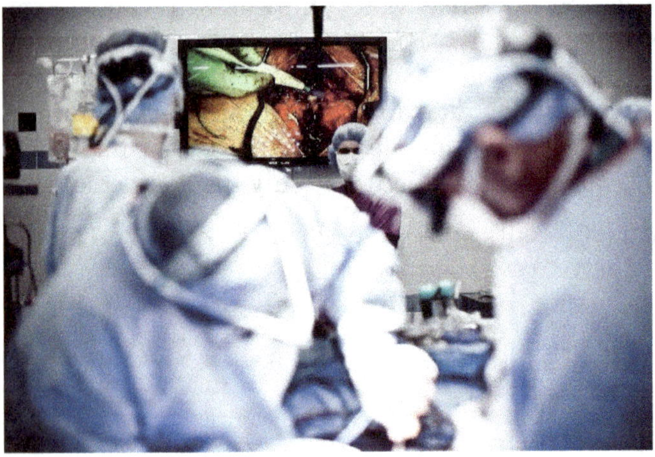

For DePuy, Zimmer, and Stryker, the advent of joint arthroplasty surgery and, later, spine fusion surgery required a fundamental change in culture and orientation from their origins as trauma companies.

While the full histories of DePuy, Zimmer, Stryker, Biomet, and the other major suppliers, as told by the people who were there, will be a future book in this series, here is a summary—perhaps a 'teaser' for what remains to be told.

DePuy

Four decades after Revra DePuy's death in 1921, surgery was becoming a standard of care and the revolution of joint arthroplasty, which would unleash a wave of innovation, more than a half a million patent filings, had fundamentally changed the business of manufacturing, marketing and logistically managing musculoskeletal tools and supplies.

DePuy, as did Zimmer and Stryker, had to re-invent itself from a splint company to a developer, educator and manufacturer of surgical instruments, implants and such adjunct products as allograft and biologic implants.

Again, like Zimmer and Stryker and, later, Biomet, DePuy initially acquired the skill sets it needed to change.

In 1968 DePuy acquired the exclusive marketing rights to Maurice Edmond Müller's hip with its 30mm head. Dr. Müller was the professor of orthopedic surgery at the University of Berne and a founder of the AO foundation—which created the modern model of surgeon training by manufacturers. To manufacture the new hip, DePuy acquired Kellogg Industries, a corset manufacturing company in Jackson, Michigan. DePuy moved its soft goods operation out of its Warsaw plant and into the Kellogg plant and converted its Warsaw facility into a hip implant manufacturing line.

In 1974, Bio-Dynamics sold DePuy Manufacturing to Boehringer Mannheim, which was owned by Corange. At the same time, DePuy Manufacturing's rival Zimmer Holdings was acquired by Bristol-Myers, an early iteration of U.S. big pharma Bristol Myers Squibb.

DePuy also began, under the leadership of Dr Charles Engh, a program to develop a cementless hip prosthesis—which achieved fixation by way of the implant/tissue interface.

Demand for hip replacements grew significantly and in 1974 and 1975, DePuy built a new 61,170 square-foot facility—then added to it over the next several years for a total of 242,110 square feet on the edge of Warsaw, Indiana.

In 1984 DePuy's president, Robert Williams, retired and James Lent, an 18-year veteran from Johnson & Johnson, became the company's new president. Lent had been president of Johnson & Johnson's orthopedic division. When he moved to DePuy, he brought with him two key JNJ senior executives—Mike McCaffrey, who had spent 14 years in sales and marketing and William Tidmore, who had run JNJ's Ethicon division for 15 years. McCaffrey became DePuy's new vice-president of marketing and sales.

Through the 1970s and 1980s, DePuy introduced a variety of hip and knee arthroplasty innovations—notably, the world's mobile artificial knee.

By 1985, when Jim Lent took the reins, DePuy's sales were $95 million.

1990s: DePuy Manufacturing Undergoes Diversification and Acquisitions

Lent and McCaffrey grew DePuy significantly through a series of acquisitions and joint ventures. DePuy's owner, Boehringer Mannheim, supported this by acquiring UK-based Thackray in 1990. The acquisition of the firm that was Charnley's original manufacturing partner, brought large joint arthroplasty distribution and sales in 100 countries worldwide to DePuy.

In 1991 DePuy purchased the Rotek Corporation, a medical products manufacturer in Albuquerque, New Mexico. DePuy's relationship with Rotek dated back to the early 1980s, when it had first hired the small company to produce a line of environmental protection products, such as face shields and gowns. After it was acquired by DePuy, Rotek expanded rapidly, moving into a new 20,000 square foot facility in 1992.

At the beginning of 1992, DePuy announced a new strategic alliance with Genentech, Inc., a San Francisco based biotechnology company. DePuy and Genentech teamed up to develop orthopedic devices that used Transforming Bone Growth Factor Beta (TGF-B), a protein that stimulated bone tissue growth and regeneration. An orthopedic device, such as a hip implant, that incorporated this protein would likely cause better growth of organic tissue and, consequently, a firmer attachment to the implant.

Also in 1992, DePuy entered the field of arthroscopy instrumentation when it acquired a 20% interest in Expanded Optics, a maker of arthroscopes. DePuy received its share in Expanded Optics when Expanded purchased one of DePuy International's subsidiaries—the Thackray-owned Scope Optics. DePuy expanded its presence in the arthroscopy market in 1993, establishing a separate manufacturing operation in Ontario, California, to produce arthroscopy instruments.

In the mid-1990s, Lent and his team made an initial foray into the spinal implant market by entering a partnership with the venerable German manufacturer

Biedermann Motech, founded in 1916. Shortly after the Biedermann Motech deal, DePuy's parent also agreed to acquire Ace Medical, a leader in the field of trauma. Finally, in 1998, Boehringer Mannheim bought the troubled spinal implant company, AcroMed for $325 million and folded it under Lent, McCaffrey, and the DePuy team.

In 1996 Lent and his team entered the sports medicine market by purchasing Orthopedic Technology, Inc., of Tracy, California. Renamed DePuy Orthotech, its products were knee braces, foot and ankle supporters, tissue fixation devices, and a full line of soft goods.

In October 1996, DePuy went public, offering 14 million shares of common stock priced at $17.50 per share. After the IPO, Corange and its subsidiaries remained the controlling stockholders. DePuy used its new public currency to, in early 1997, buy two million shares of Landanger-Camus, a leading French manufacturer of hip implants, orthopedic supplies and devices. That deal gave DePuy control of 89% Landanger-Camus and the #1 market share in France's implant market.

However, by far the most consequential event of 1997 was Roche Holding's deal to acquire DePuy's overall parent company, Corange for the tidy sum of $11 billion. The ink was barely dry on that transaction when the Roche team flipped DePuy AcroMed back to Lent's old company, Johnson & Johnson for $3.2 billion.

High finance, indeed!

The Corange acquisition closed in early 1998. It did not take but a handful of months for JNJ's purchase of DePuy to close—November 1998, in fact.

DePuy was now "DePuy, a Johnson & Johnson Company."

A few years later, DePuy sold its soft goods business.

In 2005, DePuy debuted an ostensibly longer lasting artificial surface replacement (ASR) hip acetabular system. As early as 2006, however, complaints about the implant were getting to the U.S. Food and Drug Administration. In 2009, DePuy recalled the ASR hip implant from Australia, then the rest of the world in 2010.

The issue was the ASR's metal-on-metal design. Its articulating surfaces generated metal particles leading, in some cases, to evidence of metal poisoning. Mass tort litigation reared its ugly head. In order to settle almost 8,000 ASR lawsuits, J&J and DePuy agreed in 2013 to pay $4 billion. The company also agreed to pay an additional $420 million to settle another 1,800 cases in 2015. Not all cases have been resolved as of the date of this writing.

During Lent's tenure as president, DePuy grew sales at an astonishing 20% compounded annual rate.

Zimmer

Zimmer had two interesting "firsts" in the 1950s which presaged by nearly two decades, the two most transformative events in orthopedics and spine history—joint arthroplasty surgery and spine fusion surgery.

In 1950, Zimmer was first to bring to market a hip prosthesis—a femoral only implant that had been developed by Dr. Palmer Eicher at the University of Indiana Medical Center. By 1960, Zimmer USA was the #1 supplier of implantable hip prosthetics—a very small business at the time.

In 1958, the Zimmer company also added an unusual and highly controversial new product to its line, also in the early 1950s, Dr. John Harrington's implantable rod to facilitate deformity correction and spine fusion. Harrington's rod was roundly criticized by the leading orthopedic physicians and surgeons of the day. Indeed, Harrington's own colleagues at Baylor College of Medicine actively discouraged residents from scrubbing in. At one surgeon society meeting where Harrington presented his rod, he was booed from the floor.

Yet, Zimmer added the Harrington rod to the product line in 1958, even though its sales were not material to the company.

Justin Zimmer, who was truly an inspired leader, and after his death in 1952 while on vacation in Florida, left behind a solid team to continue his vision of serving the orthopedic physician. Zimmer's sales were around $2 million annually in the early 1950s.

By 1960, Zimmer's annual sales were $4 million. In the late 1960s, Charnley's hip system came to market through London's Thackray, the Müller System was coming to market, Richards was introducing the Bechtol system.

By 1970, Zimmer's employee count had risen to 522 people and sales were now a whopping $27.2 million.

In 1971, Zimmer USA began experimenting with a non-cemented hip implant and introduced that year its own Charnley-type system, using a metal femoral stem with a plastic acetabular cup.

Bristol-Myers Buys Zimmer: 1970s-2000

In 1972, the third largest global pharmaceutical manufacturer, New York based Bristol-Myers, Inc., bought Zimmer and, along with Linvatec, created a medical device subsidiary business unit led by Charles Heimbold.

Even though Zimmer was now a subsidiary of a New York based drug company, the company remained solidly a Warsaw based manufacturer and continued to grow. Among its accomplishments during this period was the embrace of CAD/CAM systems which helped Zimmer shorten the new product development cycles and led to such innovations as a fully integrated modular system to replace artificial knees, in the 1980s.

Outside the U.S., Zimmer UK, which had been founded by former Zimmer salesman, Frank Saemann before World War II, was not owned by Zimmer, but rather by Saemann's company, the Orthopedic Equipment Company or OEC. Saemann copied the Zimmer product catalog page for page and reportedly even used Zimmer's catalog numbers modified only by a prefix or a suffix. This truly untenable situation was finally resolved when, in 1982, Zimmer paid $14 million to acquire OEC.

Among Zimmer's firsts during this period was the first arthroscopy tele-session that provided an educational seminar for 1,000 surgeons in 27 cities. The seminar featured a live arthroscopy surgery in real time. Zimmer's parent company, Bristol-Myers, began offering research grants under the Orthopaedic Research and Education Foundation (OREF) in 1983.

In 1990, Zimmer built its new corporate headquarters in downtown Warsaw, Indiana. Rivals DePuy and Biomet were several miles away, on the edge of town. Zimmer's location symbolized its roots in Warsaw, Indiana.

In 1995 Zimmer brought to market the NexGen® Total Knee solution which quickly becomes an industry leader for cruciate retaining, posterior stabilized and revision total knee arthroplasty (TKA).

In 1997, Ray Elliott joined the Zimmer team as its president. Elliott had previously been a vice-president at Bristol-Myers Squibb and brought to Zimmer 20 years of orthopedic industry experience from such firms as Baxter International, Southam, Inc., and Cablecom, Inc.

Ray Elliott would prove to be a transformative leader for Zimmer.

In 1998, under Elliott's leadership, Zimmer's sales topped $861 million, and by 1999, that number had increased to $939 million. Zimmer now employed more than 3,200 people and was closing in on $1 billion in sales.

The business of orthopedic instruments and implants is substantially different from pharmaceuticals. Elliott and his team were increasingly frustrated within the Bristol-Myers corporate umbrella. By 2001, 28% of Bristol-Myer's revenues were coming from non-pharma activities like Zimmer and Linvatec.

To get back to their knitting, the company announced that Zimmer, Linvatec and a separate consumer products division would be sold or spun off.

Elliott and his team did not want a new owner. They wanted to run the show at Zimmer.

Zimmer Holdings Is Spun Off and Goes Public

On August 7, 2001, Zimmer Holdings was officially spun off from its parent company, Bristol-Myers Squibb, and began trading on the New York Stock Exchange under the symbol, ZMH.

For three decades, Zimmer had been subsumed into Bristol-Myers. But now, under Ray Elliott the company was free to chart its own direction in the dynamic orthopedic industry of 2001.

"We are excited about the opportunity to operate Zimmer as an independent public company and to continue to strengthen Zimmer's position as a global leader in orthopedics," Elliott said at the time.

Among the benefits was that Elliott was able to significantly strengthen Zimmer's network of distributors around the world. To this day, the Zimmer distribution network that Elliott and his team built is legendary.

In 2003, Zimmer entered a bid to acquire the Swiss company Zurich, Switzerland base Centerpulse, with a U.S. headquarters in Austin, Texas. Centerpulse had a solid joint arthroplasty line but, perhaps as importantly, had a strong spinal implant and instrument line with a range of interbody and traditional hook and rod implants.

Countering Zimmer's bid for Centerpulse was London based Smith & Nephew which owned Richards Manufacturing in Memphis and was one of the top suppliers of orthopedic products in the world.

Zimmer ultimately prevailed and acquired Centerpulse in a stock and cash transaction worth $3.22 billion.

Biomet

Dane Miller had a dream while sailing with his buddy, Jerry Ferguson, back in 1975. He dreamed of a new way to make surgical implants. At the time such a dream must have seemed crazy, improbable, somewhere off in left field Dane believed that titanium was the most biocompatible metal available for implant devices. While working for Zimmer USA, he tried to introduce the material, but couldn't convince anyone that the body wouldn't reject the metal. So, he had a small rod implanted into his own arm.

Dane, Ferguson, Niles Noblitt, and Ray Harroff founded Biomet, Inc. in 1977. Biomet—Bio for body, met for metallurgical implants. Acting on that dream took some courage and was a family affair with the young group. Dane and his wife, Mary Louise, took a long-range view. Her father was a physician, and she knew about long hours.

As newlyweds, the couple lived in an 8-foot by 40-foot trailer. So, when they started Biomet in a converted barn in Warsaw, Indiana, the family just scaled back and lived frugally. "The children and I were willing to make any sacrifice," she said in a published interview. "We knew if we did it right, we could achieve this goal."

The group had just $725,000 of their own money, including a $500,000 loan from the Small Business Administration. They posted a $63,000 net loss the first year.

The wives took turns babysitting so they could go to the office and sweep the floors, type out invoices or answer phones. The men scrubbed toilets, picked up garbage, took orders and shipped product.

Garry England, the company's 41st employee said in a published interview, "I remember Dane doing wiring, office construction, sweeping, shoveling snow. It was a 'get-it-done' attitude that was very motivational to us (employees). In those days, you knew everybody who worked here by their first name; you knew their spouses' names and half their kids' names."

The financial risk was big, and the families put it all on the line. Dane and Mary Louise had personal guarantees of over $1 million dollars in debt and at the time had a net worth of $100,000.

Dane's Tenacity

Instead of intimidating him, the prospect of failure inspired Dane. "Webster's dictionary really should carry his picture next to 'tenacity' because Dane never gives up," Ferguson said in a published interview. "I mean he never gives up. It doesn't matter how bad things get." As a devout Presbyterian, Dane said he's not alone. "I rely on my spiritual underpinnings to keep me upright and moving forward."

"If we tried and failed, we were still young enough to pick ourselves up and try again," Dane told students at the Kelley School of Business as part of the Distinguished Entrepreneur-in-Residence Series. "You don't want to look back and say, 'I wish I'd tried.' The risk of failure for start-up companies is very high. So? You start over again."

Biomet Culture

One of the goals of the new company was to take suggestions from orthopedic surgeons and come out with improved implants faster than their big competitors. Right from the start, the priorities were: solid engineering, customer responsiveness, superior clinical results, and top-notch quality.

Dane said the company's culture was about taking a hands-on approach to their business. "Our employees get it done. There is no job at Biomet that isn't everyone's job. It's our company. As we grow larger, we don't want to drift into a habit of acting as if we're all managers, not employees or shareholders."

By early 1979 most of their seed money was gone. But the group was able to obtain $500,000 in equity from a venture capital investor and kept Biomet afloat until the first profitable year was realized in 1980 and a move into a new facility.

Dane: "They All Thought I Was Nuts"

By 1980, Biomet earned $1.1 million in net sales. The company went public in 1981, had Wall Street's attention by 1983, and in 1987, with $96.7 million in net sales, was deemed a "hot growth company." In 1984, Dane predicted Biomet would be a billion dollar company by 2000.

"They all thought I was nuts," said Dane. "How could anyone imagine by the year 2000 we'd be doing a billion dollars? And, in fact, in the fiscal year 2000, we reached a billion dollars."

There were some technology hiccups.

In 1983, came the Dermizip, which was lauded as the "sizzle" that sold the August 1983 public offering of three million shares. This product was supposed to catapult Biomet into the surgical wound closure market. So, of course, Dane had the new "attachment apparatus" used on his own arm.

But, it didn't hold. Not one to quit, Dane flew to O'Hare Airport to meet John Sheehan, M.D., the surgeon who had designed the product. There, in the hallway, Dane had the original product replaced and flew off to Europe. After ten days and no healing, he had the Dermizip removed in Sweden.

Dermizip never formally went to market and in-house it became known as "Dermiscar." Said one former team member, "I think Dane was the only person we left a scar on."

But it was also around this time that Dane had the test titanium rod removed from his arm. Histology and biocompatibility tests proved exactly what he had predicted—metallurgically, the titanium came out exactly like it went in. Dane didn't just use his own devices on himself, his grandmother, Grace Shumaker, was the first recipient of a Biomet-made artificial hip.

Dane and Mary Louise

Dane was born in Bellefontaine, Ohio. He and the former Mary Louise Schilke met as teens in Springfield, Ohio, at a swim club. They were married on February 19, 1966. They were married just nine days short of 49 years.

In the beginning the young couple moved every six weeks between Dayton, Ohio, where Miller worked, and Flint, Michigan, so he could attend General Motors Institute (now Kettering University). He followed his passion to a master's degree and, later, a Ph.D. in biomedical engineering from the University of Cincinnati.

With those credentials, the couple began his professional career at the Frigidaire Division, GMC in Dayton, Ohio, from 1964 to 1969, working as a cooperative engineering student. From 1972 to 1975 he was employed as the director of biomedical engineering at Zimmer. His responsibilities included engineering, prototype design and fabrication, as well as basic research support for all new product development programs. He was also responsible for coordinating and developing a custom and special product group, including marketing, sales, and manufacturing of custom products.

In 1993, Biomet rolled out the Maxim Total Knee System which incorporated primary, posterior stabilized and revision components with what was at the time, state-of-the-art biomaterials. It also was designed to give surgeons maximum flexibility and could be used for revision constrained knee indications.

In 1995, Biomet introduced a modular version of the Mallory-Head system for complicated femur revisions.

Fighting for the Team

By the mid-2000s, as a public company, Biomet was no longer entirely under Dane's control. In 2006, the company's board of directors suggested he retire after 28 years of service, and he did.

But Dane and Mary Louise didn't want to abandon their team members and planned a comeback.

"My wife and I talked seriously about riding off into the sunset," Dane said. "Then we started thinking about people. Biomet wasn't a company. It was a collection of very talented, very motivated, very dedicated people. And I wasn't comfortable with simply turning my back and riding off into the sunset. So, I began 'my little project' of putting together about $10 billion in capital to take the company private."

In 2007, with a consortium of private equity firms, Miller bought back Biomet for $11.4 billion, again living up to his credo of not wanting to look back and wish he'd tried. In 2014, Zimmer offered over $13 billion to acquire Biomet.

The buyback of Biomet was completed that spring with new CEO, Jeffrey Binder, taking the reins.

Seven years later, in 2014, Biomet agreed to merge with Zimmer in a transaction valued at $14 billion.

Stryker Corporation

Homer Hartman Stryker was born in Wakeshma Township, Michigan, on November 4, 1894, and graduated from Athens (Michigan) High School in 1913. He attended Western State Normal College, now Western Michigan University, graduating in 1916. After teaching in a one-room schoolhouse in the Keweenaw Bay school system in the Upper Peninsula, he enlisted in the U. S. Army and served in France during World War I.

When Stryker returned to the U.S., he realized that although he loved the teaching profession, he also had a strong desire to work with his hands. He talked with a family friend, a physician with a practice in Kalamazoo. Stryker's friend quickly realized that this bright, eager young man would be a good fit as a medical student. With his recommendation, Stryker was accepted into the University of Michigan medical school in 1919. However, he was required to pass a foreign language exam before beginning medical school, and he was not fluent enough in any foreign language to pass.

Stryker connected with Mary Jane Underwood, also an Athens High School graduate. Valedictorian of her class and the first female Athens High School graduate to attend college, she taught German and French in Belding, Michigan, after graduating from Northwestern University in 1916. She tutored Stryker, and he quickly picked up enough French to pass the medical school entrance exam.

Stryker needed additional money to attend medical school, so he taught school in Grand Ledge, Michigan, coached football, basketball, and baseball, worked as a barber, and pitched for the Grand Ledge semi-pro baseball team.

With the funds saved from two years of work, Stryker entered medical school at the University of Michigan in 1921. In addition to his studies, Stryker was the starting pitcher for the University of Michigan baseball team and led them to a Big 10 title.

Homer married Mary Jane Underwood, his former tutor, in 1924 in Marshall, Michigan. In 1925, Stryker graduated from the University of Michigan medical school, then interned at University Hospital in Ann Arbor for three years. After moving to Alma, Michigan, and working briefly at a small private hospital, they moved to Kalamazoo in 1928. He opened a general practice on the second floor of the State Theater building in downtown Kalamazoo.

Dr. Stryker served as the Kalamazoo County physician in 1929 and 1930 and practiced general medicine until 1936, when he returned to University Hospital in Ann Arbor to do a residency in orthopedic surgery. During his residency, he began working on ways to improve traditional procedures for moving immobile patients and to make patients more comfortable. Dr. Stryker completed the program in 1939 and together with his wife, returned to Kalamazoo.

Dr. Stryker went to work at Borgess Hospital as the regions only certified orthopedic surgeon. His office was on the second floor of the hospital and, in a pattern that would be repeated by innovative, ambitious surgeons throughout the rest of the 20th century, he also had a workshop in the basement.

It was in this workshop that Homer Stryker began to manufacture and sell some of his inventions. During World War II, his Wedge Turning Frame was sought after by the U.S. Army, so orders increased. Dr. Stryker hired two part-time workers and began producing Wedge Turning Frames and Walking Heels. His wife Mary Jane sewed canvas strings for the turning frames.

For a time during World War II, Dr. Stryker turned to the Kalamazoo Toy and Sled Company for help in manufacturing his frames. The company had been virtually shut down because of a lack of raw materials during the war, so they agreed to manufacture Dr. Stryker's frames.

In 1946, Dr. Stryker formed the Orthopedic Frame Company, Inc. By 1949, he had moved the company's headquarters to Alcott Street in Kalamazoo. The company's goal continued to be helping patients lead healthier, more active lives through products and services that made surgery and recovery simpler, faster, and more effective.

During the 1950s, Dr. Stryker worked on what was arguably his most famous invention—the Circ-O-Lectric Hospital Bed. An electric motor turned a bed, suspended between two wheels, to a vertical or horizontal position, as well as many positions in between. The device could be operated by the patient or a nurse.

Like the Wedge Turning Frame, this reduced the amount of time and effort required by staff to physically move patients. Patients liked the bed because it was more comfortable, and they could operate it themselves.

In 1955, Dr. Stryker's son Lee joined the company as general manager, and in 1958, sales hit $1 million. In 1964, Dr. Stryker retired from his medical practice and changed the name of the company to Stryker Corporation.

In 1969, Lee Stryker became president and chief operating officer. He served in that position until 1976, when he and his wife and two companions perished in a plane crash while on vacation in Wyoming. His children, Ronda, Patricia and Jon, were not on the plane and survived. Lee had helped boost the company to 280 employees and nearly $10 million in sales by the time of his death.

In 1977, John W. Brown was named president and CEO.

In 1979, Stryker Corporation entered the joint arthroplasty business by acquiring Osteonics Corporation.

1980, Homer Stryker died.

In 1992, Stryker put a big toe into the spinal implant business with the purchase of Dimso and their spinal fixation system.

1996 Stryker acquired Osteo SA and enters the orthopedic trauma business.

In 1998, Stryker significantly increases its presence in joint arthroplasty with the purchase of Howmedica corporation, the orthopedic division of Pfizer, for $1.65 billion. Howmedica became Stryker Orthopedics.

John Brown served as president, CEO and finally chairman of the board across a 32-year career with Stryker. Stryker's rise from a maker of hospital beds to a world-class medical technology company is largely attributable to Brown and corporate culture of excellence and integrity he fostered.

Under Brown's leadership, the company became a member of the Fortune 500, and Stryker received multiple accolades as one of the best managed and respected medical device and technology companies.

The Industry in 2023

Orthopedic and spine care is in the process, the slow process, of migrating to a 'smart', artificial intelligence, robotics and data driven future.

Orthopedics and spine today are very different from the world that was built and molded by L.D. Beard, Harry Treace, Ron Pickard, Dane Miller, John Brown, Jim Lentz, or Ray Elliott. Regulators and payers are more powerful than ever. Indeed, the orthopedic and spine implant revolution is, for all intents and purposes, over.

A digital revolution is sweeping through factories, operating rooms and in the critical academic world of clinical studies.

"Smart" surgery tools, algorithms for reading CT scans, robotic systems imbued with artificial intelligence, sensors, and the ability to learn anatomy, are beginning to define the practice musculoskeletal care.

Today's digital changes are equal to the transformation that occurred between 1960 and 2000.

The Largest Sector in Medicine

As of 2023, around the world, approximately 860,000 physicians, surgeons and other care givers treat 9 million patients for every type of musculoskeletal disorder known to man. In terms of supplier revenues, this is a $25 billion industry employing more than one million people.

Sales of products for spine surgery are the largest sector in musculoskeletal care reaching $10.2 billion in 2022.

Knee surgery product sales are next largest at $7.7 billion as of 2022.

Hips are third at $6.3 billion as of 2022. The fastest growing sector is the catch-all category of digital tools, which include surgical navigation systems, robotic assist systems, augmented reality systems and the rapidly developing field of Big Data and the related category of decision support systems for hospitals, payers, and caregivers, including physicians and surgeons.

The following table and chart provide sales by orthopedic category since 2008 and forecast to 2025.

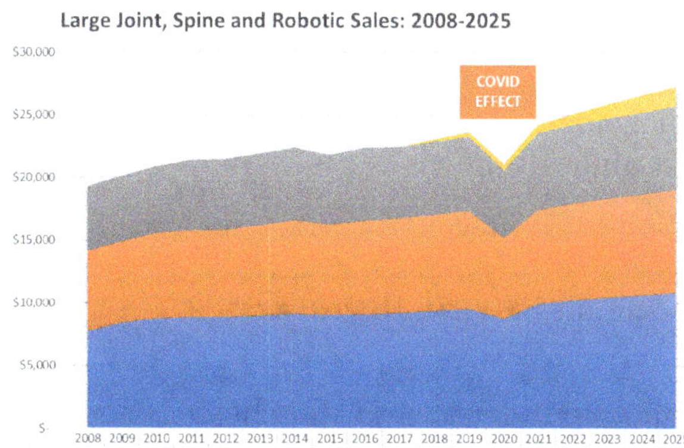

	2008	2009	2010	2011	2012	2013	2014	2015	2016	2017	2018	2019	2020	2021	2022	2023	2024	2025
Robotic System Annual Sales	$-	$-	$-	$-	$-	$-	$-	$-	$-	$-	$184	$331	$526	$667	$883	$1,13	$1.38	$1,53
Hip Annual Sales	$5,16	$5,17	$5,35	$5,61	$5.59	$5,70	$5,78	$5,54	$5,79	$5,68	$5,81	$5,90	$5,29	$6,09	$6,26	$6,40	$6,52	$6,66
Knee Annual Sales	$6,42	$6,52	$6,80	$6,91	$7.03	$7,22	$7,45	$7,24	$7,50	$7,53	$7,71	$7,85	$6,54	$7,52	$7,73	$7,90	$8,05	$8,22
Spine Annual Sales	$7,76	$8,40	$8,78	$8,88	$8,86	$8,98	$9,14	$9,06	$9,07	$9,22	$9,37	$9,53	$8,74	$9,94	$10,2	$10,4	$10,6	$10,8

EPILOGUE

The years between 1970 and 2000 are, arguably, the golden years of orthopedics and spine surgery.

It was during this period that the great leaps in hip, knee, spine, and extremity patient outcomes occurred.

It is also during this period that approximately 200,000 orthopedic and spine surgeons were trained in their craft and calling.

Jeffrey Thomas DeHaan, for example, brought orthopedic surgery to Texarkana, Texas, and served that community for 36 years.

Or, Leonard Emond, who brought hip and knee replacement surgery to Manchester, New Hampshire.

Howard Sturtz, one of the pioneers of arthroscopic surgery, treated tens of thousands of patients in San Francisco.

Victor Panitch, chief of staff at two hospitals, brought orthopedics to central Massachusetts. Ralph Gessner, in practice for 45 years, brought orthopedics to New Orleans.

Frank Trainer, chairman of St. Vincent's Department of Orthopedics and past president of the Indiana Orthopedic Society, 42 years treating patients in Indianapolis, Indiana.

Thomas Presson, 35 years serving patients in Greensboro, North Carolina.

Robert Ernest Ribbe, Vietnam Vet, 25 years in Grand Rapids, Michigan.

Jeffrey Thomas Dehaan, 36 years treating patients in Texarkana, Texas.

Norman Johanson, professor at the Lewis Katz School of Medicine and chief of orthopedics at Hahnemann

University until it closed in 2019. Thirty seven years serving patients.

Of this generation, about half (based on records we've compiled) served in the military—most in the Vietnam War.

These were the first surgeons trained in large joint arthroplasty, spine fusion, shoulder, and extremity surgery and upon whose shoulders this entire practice—the largest in medicine, serving more patients each year—was built.

This generation is also distinguished for its volunteer work.

Robert Ernest Ribbe of Grand Rapids Michigan, for example, was a member of the Christian Medical/Dental Society through which he volunteered to treat patients at no charge in Kenya, Romania, and Taiwan. He also spent almost 20 years ministering to prisoners. Dr. Ribbe and his wife extended their personal ministry to international students from Grand Valley State University.

After graduating from the University of Pennsylvania Medical School, Dr. Ribbe served in the U.S. Army, doing a residency in orthopedic surgery at Tripler Army Hospital, then a residency at Shriner's Children's Hospital in Honolulu, Hawaii and finally serving in the Vietnam war from 1968 to 1969. He was deployed to the 311th Field Hospital.

Richard Senghas, M.D., former member of the Editorial Board for the *Journal of Bone & Joint Surgery*, brought the practice of orthopedic surgery to Worcester, Massachusetts. He would eventually serve as president of the medical staff at Framingham Union Hospital and clinical instructor at the University of Massachusetts Medical School in Worcester.

After more than 30 years treating orthopedic patients, Dr. Senghas "retired" and entered Pope St. John XXIII

National Seminary, served as chaplain intern at Wellesley College and Central Main Medical Center and at age 70, in 1998, was ordained Catholic priest for the Diocese of Maine.

There are thousands more examples.

In 2022: Dr. Senghas died at age 94. Dr. Ribbe died at age 83. Dr. Johansen died at age 72. Dr. DeHaan died at age 66. Dr. Edmond died at age 93, De. Sturtz died at age 87, Dr. Trainer died at age 82, Dr. Panitch died at age 90, Dr. Gessner died at age 85 and Dr. Presson at age 82.

The first generation of orthopedic and spine surgeons is passing.

Many more of these essential stories will be told in a separate book in this series about the history of modern orthopedic and spine surgery.

The American Academy of Orthopaedic Surgeons is the principal society for orthopedic and spine surgery (the North American Spine Society—was, during its formative years, part of the AAOS). Since its founding in 1933, it has provided educational and other resources to continuously teach the practice of healing musculoskeletal injuries and disease.

AAOS membership statistics offer a glimpse into the formative, growth, and mature periods of musculoskeletal medicine.

Founded in 1933 at Northwestern University in Chicago by Willis Campbell, M.D., Edwin W. Ryerson, M.D. Fredrick J. Gaenslen, M.D.; Melvin S. Henderson, M.D.; Philip Lewin, M.D.; E. Bishop Mumford, M.D.; and H. Winnett Orr, M.D., the young organization grew from a small, barely 20 member society to 863 members over the next 12 years.

Between 1945 and the late 1960s, AAOS settled into a steady, 7% or 8% annual membership growth rate—which reflected the rapid acceleration of new knowledge and treatment strategies.

Between 1970 and 1980, AAOS membership exploded as more and more surgical residents were choosing the musculoskeletal specialty and joint arthroplasty was revolutionizing care. Also, Medicare had been passed in 1965, which funded an explosion of new patients.

Over the 1970s decade, AAOS membership grew 11% per year, on average—nearly tripling the size of the society from 5,011 members to 14,565 members.

From 1980 to 2020, membership in AAOS grew 2-3% annually. AAOS is now the largest musculoskeletal medical society in the world with approximately 39,000 members.

Since 1980, the faster growing surgeon societies have been essentially, sub-sectors of general orthopedics including, for example, societies for spine minimally invasive surgeries of all types, disc arthroplasty, scoliosis, cartilage repair, regenerative medicine, hip, knee, trauma and sports.

END OF BOOK ONE:

Healing:

The Roots of Modern Orthopedic and Spine Surgery

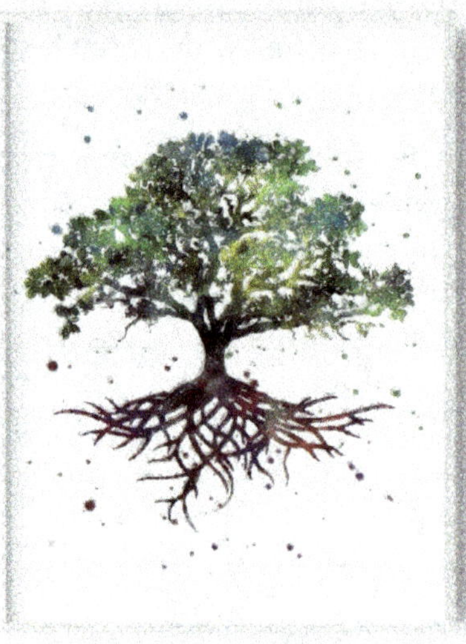

About the author: Robin R. Young

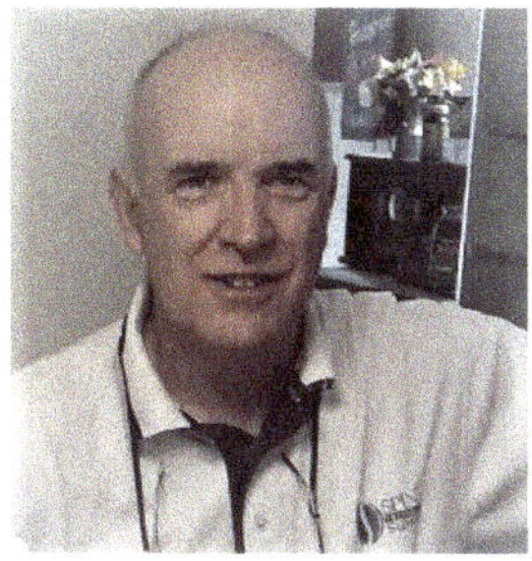

Robin Young is the founder and editor-in-chief of RRY Publications LLC, the publisher of *Orthopedics This Week*. He is also the founder of PearlDiver Technologies, Inc. a database company. Before starting his own publishing firm, Robin was an analyst and managing director for several Wall Street firms including Piper Jaffray, Stephens and HealthPoint Capital. For several years he was a member of the adjunct faculty for the Carlson School of Business at the University of Minnesota and the University of Saint Thomas. In the 1990s, he took a break from Wall Street to start a company named Clean Green Packing which invented the first starch based packing peanut. He has written thousands of articles, a handful of books, written, filed and received a patent for the use of amniotic fluid to treat knee arthritis and speaks at several medical meetings each year. He was born in Guatemala City, Guatemala and grew up in Cali, Columbia, Urbana, Illinois, Gallup, New Mexico and Canton, Ohio. Robin lives with his wife just outside of Portland, Oregon on the edge of the Willamette Valley and is usually in Sapporo, Japan for two to three months each year. He can be reached at robin@ryortho.com.

www.ingramcontent.com/pod-product-compliance
Lightning Source LLC
LaVergne TN
LVHW052244200926
848481LV00002B/272